KETO BREAD

*Ketogenic Diet to Lose Weight Including
Easy Low-Carb and Gluten-Free: Preparing
Pizza, Muffin, Biscuits and More*

Enric Scott

itional rights reserved.

Furthermore, the information that can be found within the pages described forthwith shall be considered both accurate and truthful when it comes to the recounting of facts. As such, any use, correct or incorrect, of the provided information will render the Publisher free of responsibility as to the actions taken outside of their direct purview. Regardless, there are zero scenarios where the original author or the Publisher can be deemed liable in any fashion for any damages or hardships that may result from any of the information discussed herein.

Additionally, the information in the following pages is intended only for informational purposes and should thus be thought of as universal. As befitting its nature, it is presented without assurance regarding its prolonged validity or interim quality. Trademarks that are mentioned are done without written consent and can in no way be considered an endorsement from the trademark holder.

CONTENTS

INTRODUCTION

Health-related complications such as obesity, hypertension, and diabetes have encroached into the whole world, threatening every soul across the universe. People are suffering at an alarming rate because of something they could easily control. Cases of erratic blood sugar levels have caused jitters for decades now. We are living in a world where our lifestyle dictates our mode of eating. Most people will get indulged not only in junk food but also to those types of diets which have enough meat supply. In the current generation, people consume food with high carb quantity, high levels of protein, among others.

Surprisingly, meat is consumed not because of its nutritional value but because of a culture that is slowly cropping and changing the way we live. Have you ever wondered why our great grandfathers lived for many years? Have you ever asked yourself why issues of obesity were never a problem in the past? These are specific scenarios that have left each one of us in a state of confusion. But what next? We have several issues that we can establish in our life to get rid of the problems.

Thankfully, the keto diet came to our rescue, especially those who would like to continue consuming the foods we consume every day without packing in the calories. In this book, we are going to dwell much on the bread diet since more than 80% of the total world population depends on bread. Bread has been seen as a significant source of energy for some time now. Most people depend on bread for their day to day source of nutrition, energy, and even vitamins. The rise in weight among the bread consumers is an awake up call that needs not only our attention but a quick solution. With the keto diet, however, bread can be consumed healthily.

Unfortunately, in most cases, gaining weight leads to poor body image, which has a severe feeling resulting in cases of depression. More so, you get sandwiched in between eating the bread or stopping it forever. However, as long as you feel agitated and it won't kill you, you can desert your mode of eating and look for the best diet of bread. Nevertheless, many people fear change, even though in a crucial situation like this, change is inevitable. It is because of all these reasons that I'm glad to introduce you to keto bread. It is good to note that the purpose of this keto bread is to help in losing weight.

In the next chapters, across the whole book, we are going to see much about Keto bread. You will be able to know how Keto bread uses low carb flours and sweeteners. We discuss a wide variety of Keto bread, including fat bombs such as spicy fat bombs, almond-coconut, and fat cheese bombs, among others. In other chapters, you will be able to take a look at the various buns that include fluffy keto buns, which are widely used to provide energy and has a low carb level. We also have keto burger buns, which are very nutritional and sweet. More so, they are preferred among the youths, which cover a larger percentage of the population. We also have cookies and rolls with low carbs and high-fat content. Then there are muffins and donuts which will make your day.

All in all, keto bread has got various benefits, which make it outdo other types of bread. With keto bread, issues of losing weight will never be a problem. The bread has a way of destroying fats within our bodies, which will later lead to shedding off some weight. Reducing weight improves the general body composition hence creating confidence. The diet has been proven to increase lean body mass. Fortunately, it helps people to grow leaner. A good body can then be realized when you pair this diet with strength lifting and training. Keto bread will help you to increase your energy levels.

Many people across the world require energy for daily activities. However, they will always depend on white bread, which tends to offer energy but with low nutritional value. Again, you will realize that people consume white bread because of its color and not because of the value it brings to us. Eating lots of carbs creates an imbalance situation of up and down in the level of blood sugar. However, with keto bread, the formation of energy will tend to remain constant since there is no imbalance of blood sugar level. Remember, keto bread provides energy through the oxidation of fats and not carbs. Therefore, because of this, you will be able to experience an endless supply of energy throughout the day.

Many are having various complications that are not only affecting their normal health but also inducing low self-esteem within them. Cases of lousy skin, which smells and full of acne, have so far affected the larger percentage of people. Keto diet has the power to solve this problem, and because of that, we should struggle as hard as possible to maintain the supply of this bread. Remember, keto bread will cut off the level of carbs and also deletes the issues of processed foods in your bread diets. In this case, you will realize that your gut health improves and, more so, extends to an improvement on your skin.

People are also struggling with the increased bad cholesterol level within their blood system. Many have resorted to the use of several medications without changing their bread diets. They have persistently increased their usage of white bread without understanding that processed food has a negative impact on their lives. In a quick view of solving this problematic catastrophe, many researchers have found that keto bread can enhance healthy cholesterol levels while on the other hand, eliminating the bad cholesterol. We explore this possibility in detail in the book, as well.

Besides, we have pressure in our blood system that affects each one of us day in day out. Blood pressure has been seen as a common threat not only to older people but the young generation who fails to adhere to the good eating habits. Therefore, there is a quick need for the induction of a low carb diet in our daily meal plans. A good example will be keto bread, which has a deficient level of carbs with a high content of fats. Remember, fats in keto diets are specifically for the release of energy. The fats are oxidized within the body tissues, and in the end, energy is realized. Again, when our bodies burn fats, our weight reduces. Therefore, in the end, you will have a lean body, low blood pressure, and good skin with no; acne and bad smells.

Keto bread provides a foundation in our life where we are able to fight off the problems caused by fat molecules. What you need to know is the excess level of carbs causes those fat molecules in our diet. In this case, our bodies convert excess carbs into triglycerides. Excess triglycerides come as a result of high consumption of diet full of carbohydrates and other simplest forms of starch, such as fructose. However, the introduction of the keto diet, such as bread, will help us fight off the current situation in our blood system. Remember, you need to know those fat molecules such as the ones mentioned above have health-related issues, which might cause a grave complication in our life.

A heart attack is a pertinent health issue. Many people with high reputations have succumbed to a cruel death in the hand of heart diseases. Eating white bread and other diets that have a high content of carbs, proteins, and fats have proved to be the leading cause of all these complications. In this case, the body will tend to use only carbs to provide the energy required by the body. The level of amino acids within the body will increase within the body system. In the end, causing much pain and hurting our kidneys. The fat levels will also increase within our body, which will later get their way to major organs such as hearts and kidneys. All these have been life-threatening complications that needed an immediate answer and solution. It is through this that we have come up with this book about keto bread to instill in you enough information to handle this situation.

Therefore, in this situation, keto bread has got a low carbs level diet, which helps reduce the effect of visceral fat found under the skin within the abdominal cavity. However, in the long term, fewer carbs diet in the case of keto bread will help to reduce instances of heart disease and also type 2 diabetes.

Since keto bread has got almost all the solutions to your health-related situations, I would recommend it to everyone in your household. However, you need to know that this bread has a long term benefit when you incorporate it in your diet, maintain it. Therefore, in the various chapters, I am going to dig deep on the issues that I have clearly stated here. All in all, it is now up to you to swing into action and reduce your weight as quick as possible!

CHAPTER 1: WHAT IS KETO DIET?

Life has become unbearable in many occasions where people are using white bread. That's a more refined and processed white bread. To many, it is not about the nutritional value, but the physical appearance such as its colors and how it pleases the eyes. White bread has led to life-threatening complications stemming from heart diseases to poor body image. Poor body image comes as a result of obesity. Due to this, there is an urge to introduce a diet which will help to solve all the issues affecting our life. The diet should comprise of a low level of carbs, fewer proteins, and normal level of fats.

Fortunately, the ketogenic diet suits all the above. In a quick view, we can deduce that the keto diet is a diet comprising of very low carb and a high level of fat. Meaning, incorporations of this diet into our body system will result in the assimilation of excess fats as compared to the carbs. Therefore, our blood system and our muscles will end up with a high-fat level. The keto diet, which is also known as ketogenic, shares several similarities with the likes of low carb diets and Atkins diets.

Keto diet involves the process of reducing the intake of carbohydrates while on the other hand, increasing the fat intake. In this case, your body is continuously undergoing crucial metabolic changes resulting in what we call ketosis. Therefore, the ketosis process will ensure that your body can burn fats and oxidize them to release energy. From our perspective, especially from the layman's language, we are much aware of the function of carbs in our body system. That's, they play a significant role in the production of energy.

However, this has never been efficient in solving the issue of body weight. Remember, you should know that the main aim of introducing the ketogenic diet is to help us in solving the obesity problems. White bread with a high level of carbs will never solve this. Therefore, in this ketosis process, fats are turned into ketones. All these take place within the liver. It is from the liver that we are able to have energy that the brain normally uses.

The ketogenic diet can tremendously reduce both the insulin and blood sugar levels. Fortunately, these plus increased ketones within the liver have various health benefits. There are several types of ketogenic diets that I am going to list down in point form. But you have to make sure that you follow a good guideline on how to implement each one of them.

Different Types of Keto Diets

1. Targeted keto diet
2. Cyclical keto diet
3. The high protein keto diet
4. Standard keto diet

In a summary of the various forms of keto diets, you will realize that the targeted keto diet will allow you to introduce more carbs in the diet. However, this is during exercises and workouts only. On the other hand, cyclical requires a clear follow up of the alternate implementation of the ketogenic diets and high carb diets. In this case, you will have to assimilate keto diet for the first 5 days in a week then followed by the 2 days specifically for high carb diets.

Moreover, there is a standard diet that comprises of low carb level, high fat diet plus a moderate protein level — the standard consists of 20% proteins, 75% fats, and 5% carbs. We also have a high protein keto diet, which is somehow similar to the standard keto diet. In this diet, there is more protein, which marks the difference between the standard diet and the high protein keto diets. More so, this diet consists of 5% carbs, 35% proteins, and 75% fats.

As earlier been said, keto diet consists of a diet comprising of high-fat level, low carb intake, and moderate protein. You can clearly conclude that the diet can help us solve various problems facing us in life. The issues include obesity, diabetes and prediabetes, heart diseases, cancer, and much more. Below are some of the beneficial functions of keto diets;

- Keto diet reduces weight

The ketogenic diet can help you lose weight.

Moreover, it helps in lowering risks, especially the ones that result in various diseases. Ketogenic involves the oxidation of excess fats in our body to release energy, which is being used by different body organs such as the heart, lungs, and even brains. The excess fats are the ones that are always responsible for the increase in weight. Again, weight also comes as a result of a high intake of carbohydrates in our diets.

However, in this diet, it involves the intake of low carbs. In the end, this will lead to the loss of weight, thus improving the overall body image. Apart from losing weight, this diet helps in improving the cholesterol and insulin levels in the blood system. People placed or maintaining this diet are capable of losing weight three times more than those placed under the recommended diet by the professionals. The ketogenic diet also provides a situation where your body will incorporate more protein.

Protein forms parts of the bodybuilding aspect of our system. Again, protein is useful since they act as a protective mechanism to our body. Apart from this, protein helps in restoring our body functions. Most damaged parts of our bodies are prepared with the help of different types of proteins within our bodies. However, this is only possible with the help of body organelles such as lysosomes and ribosomes. In the liver, there is the formation of ketones, which help in lowering the blood sugar levels. Also, it improves insulin sensitivity.

- The diet reduces diabetes and prediabetes

Diabetes involves various changes, especially in high blood sugar, metabolism, and insulin malfunctions. Losing fat through a keto diet will help reduce the chances of getting type 2 diabetes. Again, cases of metabolic syndrome and prediabetes always come as a result of excess fats within our bodies. Therefore, when the body burns excess fats, it will be preventing all these health-related complications.

Other benefits of keto diet which are health-related

From the beginning, the keto diet was mainly to treat diseases such as neurological illness. A good example included epilepsy. However, many studies have now indicated that the keto diet has various benefits in managing different conditions that are related to our health. These health conditions include:

Epilepsy: several studies have shown that this diet can reduce the effects of seizures in children who have epilepsy.

Cancer: the keto diet is being deployed and implemented in various treatments involving several types of cancer. Again, it helps in slowing the growth of tumors within our bod

Heart-related diseases: keto diet helps in improving the blood sugar level, reducing the bad cholesterol, and also lowering the blood pressure. In the end, heart attack cases will never be an issue.

Alzheimer's disease: the diet is capable of slowing the progression rate of Alzheimer's disease and also reducing its symptoms.

Acne: this is a skin disease that comes as a result of eating too many sugars and highly processed food. However, with the keto diet, the level of insulin within our blood system will reduce. More so, you will be eating food that's not processed. Again, with the keto diet, you will be experiencing fewer sugars in your diet.

Parkinson's disease: the diet helps in improving the symptoms of the disease. As a result, you will be controlling the disease in a more manageable way.

Brain injuries: brain injuries are caused by hitting and other accidents. The keto diet is capable of reducing concussions and sometimes can even help in the recovery of the brain.

There is also polycystic ovary syndrome: The ovary is always affected by the level of insulin within our body. This syndrome tends to reduce in conditions where the blood sugar level is low. Again, it will also decrease in a situation where insulin within our bodies reduces.

Keto Flu

The keto diet is gaining popularity and becoming famous not only to older people but also to the youths. Its main objective in helping with weight loss, treatment of health-related diseases such as blood pressure, preventing other conditions such as acne has made it well-known across the globe. However, changing into a diet, you were never used to is not easy. That's, indulging in a keto diet has got some side effects that you need to take care of so that you realize its full effectiveness. As mentioned earlier, the keto diet consists of intake of low carbohydrates, high level of fats, and also moderate protein. While this diet is regarded as safe for many people, it is associated with some side effects which are not good at all. All these side effects combine to make up what we can now refer to as keto flu. Therefore, Ketu flu refers to the general terms of total symptoms someone experiences while using the keto diet for the first time.

Keto diet has got side effects, just like other diets. Sometimes back, you would wish to indulge in other diets such as vegan diet and so on. The same affects you will experience there are the same in this situation. Always our bodies react to new changes. In most cases, these changes might affect us positively, while sometimes, we might have a negative impact on our side. In this case, the body is getting inducted into the keto diet, which comprises of low carbs and high intake of fats. Again, the level of protein slightly increases. This implies that the body will start surviving on a low level of carbohydrates, thus prompting the body to react in this way.

When you reduce the level of carbs within your diet, the body system is forced to use ketones during oxidation to release energy. That's starch related products such as glucose, carbohydrates, and fructose will never have a purpose in your body. Remember, ketones are by-products that come as a result of the breakdown of excess within our body tissues. In this case, this fat breakdown leads to the formation of energy which the body requires for various physiological and biological activities. Usually, fat forms the secondary source of fuel, especially when the starch related products such as glucose is not available within our blood system.

Therefore, the process of burning fat in our body is what is called ketosis. In most cases, it occurs in rare circumstances, which include fasting and starvation. Also, our body can achieve this ketosis process when we adopt a diet with low carb intake. Moreover, in the keto diet, there is always a reduction of carbohydrates to almost 50 grams per day. This kind of reduction will automatically cause a greater impact on your body. As a result of this, it will lead to withdrawal-like symptoms. These symptoms resemble the ones you might experience while undergoing weaning off addictions. That's eliminating addictive substances such as caffeine, and using keto diet results in various symptoms, especially if it's your first time. Below are symptoms that are written in point form for easy understanding.

Symptoms

Changing from your diet to a new diet is a major challenge not only to your body but also to your personal life. When you abruptly stop having your usual diet with excess carbohydrates to a low carb diet, your body will entirely react. This reaction might take quite some time since the body needs to adapt entirely to this new keto diet. Unfortunately, some people may experience a lot of difficulties while, to others, challenges could be less.

Therefore, it is good to note that symptoms have no specific days. Some might appear as early as possible, while others might take quite several days. What you need to know is that in the end, these symptoms will eventually show up, and their impacts will be felt. In most cases, these symptoms can be less mild or severe, depending on the immune system of the consumer.

However, it is also good to understand that not everybody will experience the side effects of the keto diet. Some might transition very well without any problematic issues. That's not experiencing any form of symptoms. Unfortunately, some people will eventually face the wrath of transition. In this case, they will end up having the following symptoms:

- Constipation
- Headache
- Weakness
- Sugar cravings
- Irritability
- Muscle crumps

> ➤ Poor concentration
> ➤ Difficulty sleeping
> ➤ Vomiting
> ➤ Muscle soreness
> ➤ Dizziness
> ➤ Diarrhea
> ➤ Stomach pain
> ➤ Nausea

Keto diet has a challenge, which may lead to depression and stress a lot. Symptoms in new entries can be for one week; however, in some people, this might even take quite several times. At some point, you might also feel like giving up due to their distressing challenges. To avoid giving up, I have come up with clear illustrations on how to deal with the keto flu. That's to eliminate them completely.

How to Eliminate Keto Flu

The keto flue has the tendency of causing miseries in your life if not well controlled or maintained. That's being managed accordingly. Fortunately, there are various ways in which we can use to delete the keto flu and create harmony with our body once more. Moreover, this will allow our bodies to undergo the period of transition more easily smoothly. Below are several techniques you can eventually use to get rid of the Ketu flu:

Stay Hydrated: during this transition period, you should struggle to drink as much water as possible. Drinking water is helpful as it provides excess fluid within our body system.

In most cases, the oxidation of fats in our body leads to the release of water. That's, we always get ourselves sweating. Again, the introduction of the keto diet eliminates the high intake of carbohydrates. Carbohydrate plays a significant role in water storage, especially within our body. In that, glycogen always binds with water and helps in preserving a bit. When carbohydrates are eliminated or reduced, the level of glycogen plummet. In the end, the excretion of water from the body takes place.

Therefore, staying hydrated will help you solve the symptoms that are related to muscle cramps and fatigue. Again, drinking a lot of water will help you affect some symptoms related to diarrhea. It is good to understand diarrhea leads to loss of excess fluid within the body system.

Avoidance of Strenuous Exercise: exercise is essential since it helps us lose weight, stay healthy, and improves our body image. However, strenuous exercise during keto flu is dangerous. During the first week of the keto diet, you will be experiencing fatigue, stomach discomfort, and even muscle cramps. These symptoms are similar to the ones you will realize during strenuous training. Therefore, it is essential to keep your body relaxed and avoid overtraining. There are other activities such as intense biking, weight lifting, running, and even some strenuous workouts that also need to be put behind during this transition. However, avoid deserting all the exercises. In this case, some exercises help our system is working well. These include leisurely biking, yoga, and even walking.

Strive for Adequate Sleep: irritability and fatigue are always familiar to those who are undergoing the keto diet. When you don't sleep, the level of cortisol, which is a stress hormone, rises. Thus causing more damage or negative impacts on the already worsening situation. Your mood will be affected, and in the end, you will feel more stressing symptoms resulting from the diet. Therefore, sleeping is essential in your life. In case you might be experiencing a lack of sleep, you can try the following:

- Shower and take a bath more often
- Check on your caffeine intake and reduce it
- Switch off any ambient light
- Avoid oversleeping most of the time

Eat Enough Fat and fewer Carbs: transitioning is not easy, and this can make you crave some restricted foods. That's bread, cookies, bagels, and even pasta. However, to avoid these cravings, you should eat enough fat, which is provided in the keto diet and fewer carbs. In the end, you will feel satisfied. Several pieces of research show that diets with low carbs can compensate for the lack of sweets. For those people getting it worse during the transition may eliminate carbs progressively. This will create a smooth transition eventually. This implies that you will be getting into both moderate protein and high fat as you cut off carbs in your diet.

How to Get Into Ketosis

Ketosis is a metabolic process that creates various health benefits in our body. During this process, the body tends to convert fat into some compounds, which it later uses as a primary source of energy. That's, the fats are converted into useful ketones, which act as the primary source of energy as compared to the normal situation where carbs provide the necessary foundation of energy production. Several studies conducted have shown that these diets promoting the ketosis process can reduce weight. As a result, they help in solving health-related complications such as hypertension, obesity, blood sugar levels, and even a high level of insulin within the blood. More studies are indicating that the ketosis process helps in reducing the risks of getting type 2 diabetes. More so, cases of neurological disorders, among others, are eliminated.

Therefore, achieving a total state of ketosis will take quite some time. Moreover, this process will require proper planning and working on the goals to fulfill all your plans. It is good to note that achieving this is not as simple as some people might think. This is always unlike cutting the carbs level within the diet. Several useful tips will help you indulge in ketosis. These tips are proven to be very helpful, and following them will eliminate the severe effects of keto flu.

Consume less carb

Eating less carb in our diet is the best foremost way of achieving ketosis. Previously, under normal conditions, your body cells use the finest forms of starch, such as glucose, fructose, and lactose, in proving fuel. However, at some point, sources of fuel might be derived from elsewhere. In this case, fatty acids and ketones will form the other primary source of fuel. In simple terms, ketones are also known as ketone bodies. Glycogen is stored in the muscles and liver.

However, it is good to note that glycogen is glucose but in another form. Taking low carb will reduce the level of glucose within the body. Later, this will affect the level of glycogen and in the end, reduces the levels of insulin hormone. All this process allows the release of fatty acids from where they are stored. The liver will then convert fatty acids into ketones. That's ketone bodies acetone. Also, this conversion results in beta-hydroxybutyrate and acetoacetate.

Body organs such as brains make use of these ketones as a source of fuel. In this case, many people have different levels when it comes to initiating the ketosis process. Some need less than 50 grams per day, while others will require 20 grams or even less.

In short, when you limit your carb intake to a range of 20-50 grams per day, you will realize a lower insulin and blood sugar levels. This initiates the release of fatty acids, which your liver will later convert to release energy.

Introduce coconut oil in all of your diets

Coconut oil always gives a smooth initiation into the ketosis process. This is because it contains medium-chain triglycerides. This type of fats has got several benefits, which include its ability to get converted into ketones easily. Again, it is easily absorbed and taken into the liver, where it is used as a source of energy is realized. Most studies indicate that people who are suffering from diseases such as Alzheimer's need to consume a lot of coconut oil. This is extended to those suffering from neural disorders — the most profitable type of MCTs the lauric acid.

Lauric acid contains about 50% of fats. Many people prefer MCTs in inducing ketosis, especially in those suffering from epileptic. In this case, carbs will still be available here. However, you should note that coconut oil has got various side effects, such as diarrhea and stomach cramping. Due to this, the addition of it into your diet should be observed with immediate care and done slowly. You can begin with one spoon per day, then graduate to two and go on with higher numbers.

Check on the levels of ketone and make adjustments.

Maintaining and achieving ketosis will be a personal contribution. That's it is like a goal you are trying to achieve. Because of that, you need to test your levels of ketone and add where possible continually. By doing this, you will be achieving your goal. You can always use your urine, blood, or breath to test for the three types. That's acetoacetate, beta-hydroxybutyrate, and also acetone. Several studies indicate you can use your breath to measure the levels of acetone in your body. This process will help you to keep track of the ketosis process, especially on those who are undergoing the ketogenic diet.

Control your protein intake

The process of ketosis requires a moderate protein intake. That's neither excess nor less. In epilepsy patients, ketone levels are maximized through the intake of restricted protein and carbs. Cancer patients, too, require the same diet since it reduces the growth of the tumor. Even though this is useful, but many people find it weird for the sacrificing protein to realize a high level of ketones. This is because, in most cases, proteins produce amino acids in our bodies. These amino acids are the main source of the gluconeogenesis process. Here, your liver can supply glucose for the cells such as red blood cells and some organs which cannot use ketones as fuel. These organs include portions of the brain and kidneys.

Again, you should take a high level of protein to maintain the mass of the muscles, especially when the intake of carb is deficient. More so, during exercise, especially for weight loss, your protein intake should be high. Therefore, excessive consumption of protein leads typically to a reduction in ketone while other the other hand, you might experience loss of muscle mass when you consume very little protein. Due to this, there is a need to control your protein intake.

Notes: Other ways can help you get into ketosis. Checking on your physical activities can greatly help in getting into the ketosis. We also have a fasting process and increasing your fat intake.

Products Allowed On Keto Diet

Many people are turning into a ketogenic diet at an alarming rate. This popularity is caused by its usefulness in solving various health-related complications. However, some products are allowed while some are not. In this topic, we are going to take a look at what we should eat in the ketogenic diet.

- Seafood: seafood such as fish and shellfish are always keto-friendly. We have salmon which provide the diet with vitamin B, selenium, and even potassium. Therefore, seafood has no carbohydrates, or some consist of less carb. The presence of excess omega -3, minerals, plus vitamins makes this diet acceptable. Also, try as much as possible to have two servings per week.
- Fewer carb vegetables: some non-starchy vegetables contain low calories and carbs. However, they are highly nutritious with excess vitamin C and other minerals. Therefore, most non-starchy veggies have a net carb of about 1-8 grams. They are much allowed in the diet. Again, they are versatile, nutritious, and

can help in eliminating risks related to diseases.

- Cheese: most cheese is both delicious and nutritious. All types of cheese are low in carbs with a high level of fats. All these nutritional values make them fit in the keto diet. They are also rich in calcium and proteins.
- Avocados: all types of avocados are healthy and always recommended for consumption. They have about 2 grams of carbs in every serving. They also contain several nutrients, such as potassium. Avocados can improve heart-related complications. More so, avocado possesses a high level of fiber.
- Poultry and meat: these staple foods in the keto diet. They lack carbs and always rich in vitamins B. also, they contain various minerals such as zinc, selenium, and even potassium. Moreover, they are the primary source of high-quality protein. Remember, proteins play a significant role in feeding up the muscle mass, especially during a low carb diet. Animals feeding on grass have the best meat ever. That's, their meat contains a high level of omega -3 fats, antioxidants and also conjugated linoleic acid.
- Eggs: they are believed to be the healthiest food on the planet and also the most versatile ingredients in your diet. They possess less carb and have the ability to maintain you full for several hours. Eggs are high in nutrients, and because of these, they can eliminate risks related to heart complications. Fortunately, eggs can also help in eye treatment.
- Coconut Oil: coconut oil has some properties that suit it in the ketogenic diet. All types of coconuts possess MCTs, which increases the production of the ketone. More so, coconut oil can promote the burning of the belly fat hence leading to loss of weight. Again, it can increase the metabolic rate of the body.
- Cottage cheese and plain Greek yogurt: these are

healthy food with high protein content. They always reduce appetite and increases fullness in most of the time.

- Olive Oil: it has beneficial attributes, especially to the heart. It is suitable for salad dressings. Also, you can add it to cooked foods.
- Nuts and Seeds: they help in eliminating risks that are related to heart complications. Also, they are high in fiber.
- Berries: they are highly nutritious and eliminate the risks of diseases.

Products to Avoid

Any form of food that is having lots of carbs should be avoided in the keto diet. Below is a list of some of the foods you can eventually do away with or just reduce them completely:

- Unhealthy fats such as processed oils from vegetables
- Legumes or beans such as peas, chickpeas, lentils, and even kidney beans
- Starches or grains which include pasta, cereal, or even wheat-based products.
- Sugary foods such as soda, smoothies, cakes, candy, fruit juice, ice cream, and so on.
- Diets with low-fat content such as the ones with highly processed carbs and much more.
- Some sauces or condiments contain much sugars and fats which are unhealthy.
- Alcohol should not be in your diet since they contain high carb
- Tubers and root vegetables such as potatoes, carrots or even parsnips

References

Kubala, J. (2018, April 3). The Keto Flu: Symptoms and How to

Get Rid of It. Retrieved from https://www.healthline.com/nutrition/keto-flu-symptoms

Mawer, R. (2018, June 30). The Ketogenic Diet: A Detailed Beginner's Guide to Keto. Retrieved from https://www.healthline.com/nutrition/ketogenic-diet-101

Palsdottir, H. (2017, June 3). What Is Ketosis, and Is It Healthy? Retrieved from https://www.healthline.com/nutrition/what-is-ketosis

CHAPTER 2: LOW CARB FLOURS AND SWEETENERS TO USE WHILE BAKING BREADS

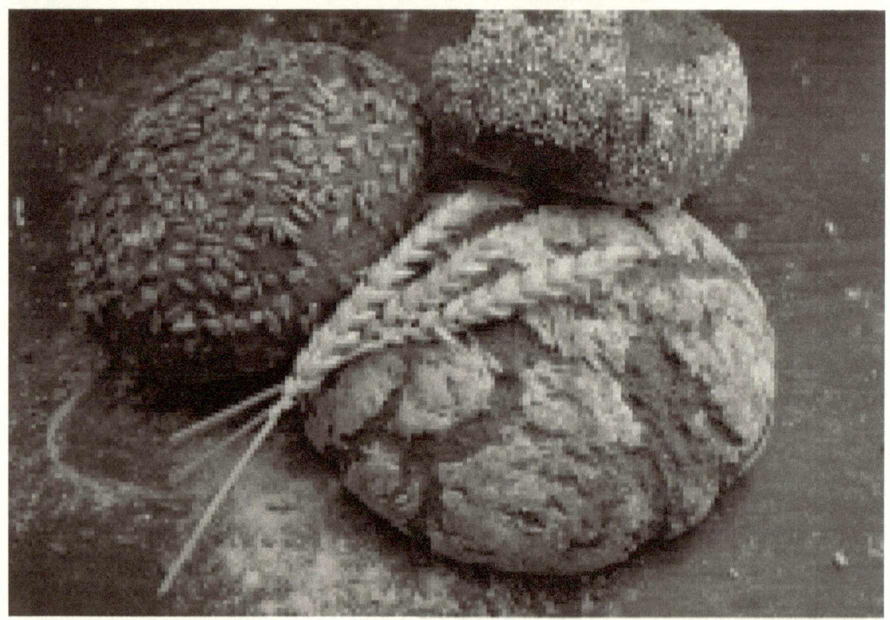

Getting the correct low carb flour when you are baking, especially in Keto diet is always a challenge. Also, finding a low carb flour that you can use as replacements to yield bread, cakes, cookies, and even pancakes still prove to be a significant challenge. Therefore, with the current situation, you realize that wheat flour and its constituents are highly processed hence, making them inappropriate for the ketogenic diet. In wheat, just a quarter of a cup has almost 22 grams of carbs. In this case, it cannot be suitable for the ketogenic diet. As a result of these, we have come up with the best low carb flours and sweeteners that you can use in baking in a keto diet, as shown below.

The below are highly appropriate in this diet, and their storage should be taken with great care. That's, they should be stored in airtight containers to avoid any reactions between the air particles with the various low carb flours.

Various types of Low Carb Flours

Coconut flour

Coconut flour has multiple benefits when it comes to health issues. The flour is everywhere, and in most occasions, many of us consume it every day. Coconut flour is the best replacements for cakes, muffins, and even brownies recipes. Fortunately, we prefer this when we are looking for a consistency moist in our keto diets. We always prefer this flour due to its low carb content. Remember, it is a low carb count and not a no carbohydrate.

In every diet, even in the ketogenic diet, you can't completely cut off the supply of carb since all these have various functions in the bodies. That's, they not only help in the production of energy but also assists in other factors such as body mass and much more. Coconut flour forms a better foundation that suits in the keto diet. The main advantage of coconut flour is its ability to withdraw moist from other ingredients such as water and eggs in the making the whole diet to that consistency in terms of moisture.

Coconut flour attribute or traits that enable it to absorb moisture, has given the ketogenic diet a new look, especially in the sectors of muffins and other keto products. That's, it can prevent it from drying. Due to all these, people are narrowed and closed in a world of confusion and are unable to identify them unless they are informed. Examples of coconut flour recipes, especially in keto diet include the following:

1) Chocolate muffins which are within the keto diet
2) Peanut butter, that's, choc chic blondies types

    3)   Cheesecake, that's low carb swirl brownies.

Nutrition of the coconut flour will include the following:
Two tablespoons will have the following;
Calories------------------- 45
Net carbs----------------- 3 grams
Fiber---------------------- 8 grams
Proteins------------------ 4 grams

Almond flour

You can use this for low carb crusts and keto cookies. Almond flour, low-carb wheat flour substitute for Keto cookies. It is essential in the preparation of dessert recipes and other baking purposes. You can prepare almond flour by grinding the blanched almonds and remember to remove the skin. It is also a versatile ingredient, and because of this, it is the primary source of flour within all the keto recipes.

Therefore, the flour will work very well in all baking, which includes keto baking for cookies. It is also a long-lasting flour. That's, it can last for over seven months when kept in an airtight container. Also, make sure that this container is well maintained in the refrigerator. The following are examples of different recipes where you can use almond flour.

1)   Keto bread
2)   Dairy-free vanilla with coconut
3)   Low carb cherry with cream chocolate cookie bars
4)   Fried chicken that's southern keto chicken
5)   Savory and a low carb parmesan pie crust

Almond flour consists of the following:
A quarter cup will have the following;
Fats--------------------------- 14 grams
Proteins------------------------6 grams
Net carbs----------------------3 grams

Almond meal

In this flour, you make it without removing the skin of the almonds. That is, you grind almond with its skin so that it is more course as compared to the almond flour. In most cases, you can use almond meal in making low carb cookies in the keto diet and also while preparing pie bases. Almonds are easy to make. You can prepare some of it by using even a blender, but make sure the almonds you are using are unsalted. Therefore, below are some of the recipes where you can easily apply the almond meal.

Macadamia nut cookies which are low carb
Bacon muffins and sour cream (low carb)
Key lime pie (low carb)
Nutrition of almond meal
A quarter cup will have the following;

Fat----------------------------------14 grams
Protein------------------------------- 6 grams
Fiber--------------------------------- 3 grams
Net carbs----------------------------- 3 grams

Ground flaxseed

It is also known as flax meal. Also, this flour is a good substitute in several recipes involving low carbs baking. In situations, you use it instead of eggs. Therefore, you can use flaxseed in the case where some people are allergic to eggs and also when some are observing a vegetarian meal plan. That's, they are not eating animals and their products. It is very nutritious and healthy. It is known to contain omega -3 elements and several vitamins such as vitamins B. also it consists of several essential fatty acids that the body usually requires. Like any other flour, you should make sure flaxseed is kept in an airtight container. Remember, this flour is very unstable. It gets unusable very quickly. The following is one of the recipes where flaxseed is applicable.

➤   Flaxseed crackers

The nutrition of flaxseed contains:

2 tsp. Contains the following;

Net carb--------------------------------- 1 gram

Calories-----------------------------------72

Proteins--------------------------------- 3 grams

Fiber------------------------------------- 4 grams

Psyllium husk

It helps in the substitution of the keto flours. Psyllium husk adds up to the various low carb flours already found within the ketogenic diet. In most cases, people use it for toppings, especially from cereal purposes. Also, you can use it as a primary source of dietary fiber. However, in keto cooking where the low carb is applicable, it fits very well. This is because of its low carb contents. Fortunately, apart from its usage as a low carb component in the flour category, psyllium husk contributes much in the gut health. That's, it has excellent characteristics of prebiotic.

It also provides a good substitution in places where eggs are applicable, and moistness is also required. All in all, it can also be applied where no carb is needed at all. Psyllium husk is always a good source of fiber with a net carb count of about 1.5 grams per each tablespoon. Incorporating this flour in your keto diet helps you with several advantages. That's, you can eat your meals with correct moisture, and also, you will be in a position of assimilating lots of cheese in your body system. Remember, cheese is an excellent ingredient in the keto diet since it has got high-fat content and a high level of protein with zero carbs.

In some situations, its natural laxative character enables it to be used as a fiber supplement. However, you must note that you can only use a heavily diluted psyllium husk since assimilating it raw may lead to some difficulties, such as choking. Unfortunately, psyllium husk doesn't have many recipes like other types of flours being used in the ketogenic diet. A good example where it is applied is in the bacon rolls and keto cheese. In most cases, it is good to note that psyllium husks are majorly for increasing bulkiness some recipes while reducing the level of carbs in baking recipes. Apart from this, it is added in some bread, such as almond flour bread, to increase the moisture content. That's to prevent it from drying.

The nutrition of psyllium husks consists of the following:

18 grams of psyllium husk which is equivalent to one table-spoon consists of the following;

Fiber------------------------13.5 grams

Net carbs-------------------- 1.5 grams

Sweeteners To Use While Baking Breads

The ketogenic diet involves deleting or instead of cutting back on foods that contain high carbs levels such as desserts, starches, and processed snacks. Always this is essential to your body since the body needs to undergo ketosis process. That's, your body will start burning excess fats to yield energy instead of using carbs as its primary source of fuel. The process of ketosis creates a situation where you have to reduce the sugar intake for its to function appropriately. However, this has become one of the most significant challenges not only to older people but the whole world at large. In real life, many people are fighting off an obsession of depending too much on baked goods, sweetened beverages, dressings, and even sauces. To help cut off this, there are various sweeteners that you can use since they contain low carbs, as shown below.

Stevia

It is derived from a plant called stevia rebaudiana, and it is one of the natural sweeteners we do have. It is part of the nonnutritive sweetener since it lacks or contains less or very little carbs. In most cases, it doesn't have calories. Stevia has other health benefits since it can lower the blood sugar level. Most stevia is very sweet, and because of this, many people prefer using less of it to realize their expected flavor. That's one cup of about 200 grams of regular baking sugar that can be equivalent to only 4 grams of stevia.

Sucralose

Sucralose forms parts of the artificial sweeteners that cannot undergo metabolism. As a result, they passed through the body without being digested. Therefore, they don't contribute either calories or even carbs. Most sweeteners have a bitter taste. However, Splenda, which is part and parcel of sucralose, lacks the bitter taste. As a result, it is more popular as compared to other sweeteners. Sucralose has got a negative side effect of being affected by high temperatures. As a result, you should try to avoid it as much as possible, especially in baking recipes. However, you can use it to sweeten foods like yogurt, oatmeal. Again, you can also apply it to drinks. Surprisingly, pure sucralose is more than 600 times sweeter as compared to normal and regular sugar.

Erythritol

A type of sweetener that occurs naturally and has an alcoholic taste. It's found within the mouth and always gets detected by the receptors of the tongue. It is always not very sweet as compared to regular sugar. Its composition ranges from 5% calories to 4 grams of net carb. Due to its features, it can lower blood sugar levels, especially within the body. It has smaller particles, which makes it suitable for its functions. That's, its usage cannot lead to any digestive complications as compared to other sugar alcohols. You can use it in both cooking and baking in various recipes. However, erythritol slightly dissolves in food substances. That's, its rate of dissolving is very low as compared to regular sugar. As a result, it can create a gritty texture in most foods where it is applied.

Xylitol

Another form of sugar alcohol is xylitol. You can find this sugar alcohol in products like mints, candies, and even free gums. It is always sweet like sugar, also though it consists of 4 grams of carbs and 3 calories per gram. Xylitol's carbs don't count, and because of this, they cannot raise insulin levels or increase blood sugar levels.

Sweetener from monk fruit

It is derived from monk fruit. Monk fruit has its origin from Southern China. More so, this plant has compounds refer to as mogrosides. Mogrosides account for the sweetness of the fruit since they are antioxidants.

Yakon syrup

You can quickly obtain this from the roots of the yakon plant. Geographically, this plant is found in South America. Yakon plant contains a sweeter syrup which comprises of fructooligosaccharides. Unfortunately, your body cannot digest this type of fiber. More so, this compound consists of various sugars, which include fructose, sucrose, and even glucose. You can also apply yakon syrup in places where you don't want to use sugar. That's drinks like tea, coffee, cereal, and even in salad dressings.

References

Ditch the Carbs. (n.d.). The Ultimate Guide to Low-Carb Flours [Blog post]. Retrieved from https://www.ditchthecarbs.com/low-carb-flours/

My Keto Kitchen. (2018, October 6). Low Carb Flours – Keto Flour Substitutes for Baking – "Secrets" to Making Your Favorite Recipes [Blog post]. Retrieved from https://www.myketokitchen.com/keto-resources/low-carb-flour-alternatives-lchf-keto-cooking/

CHAPTER 3: BREAD IDEAS

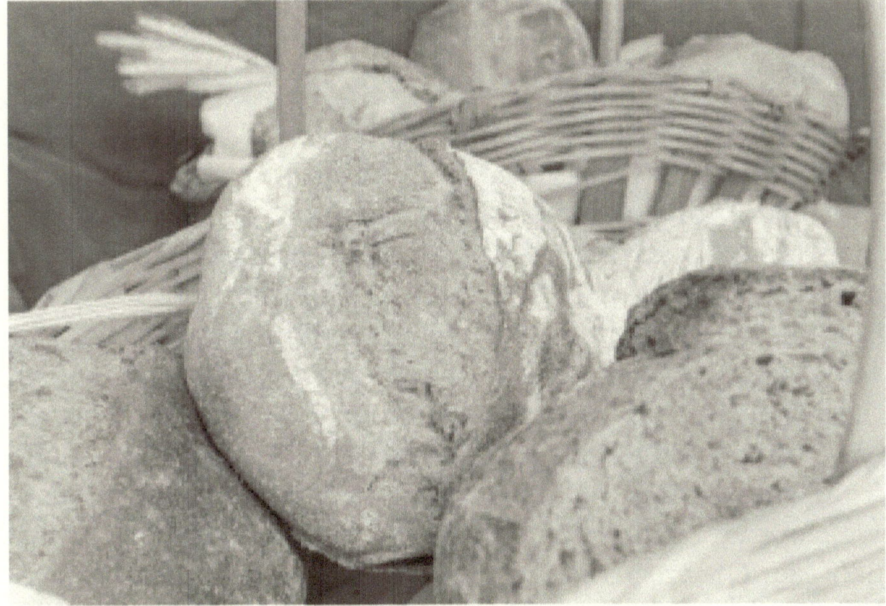

It is a well-known fact that human beings eat bread and also other kinds of grains. Most of what we eat in our diet falls into this kind of category. It includes the types of bread found in bagels, hamburgers, muffins, sandwiches, and also hotdog buns. These examples show us that we utilize wheat in most of our meals. This can be a very bad motivation killer to people who are in a low carb diet for personal reasons or medical reasons. It can also be to maintain their health and wellbeing. Anyone who wants to lose weight should not have to worry about getting rid of bread from their menu.

There are a lot of low carb kinds of food which we can use to replace bread in our routine. We do not need to worry about the alternatives for substituting our bread that is full of carbs. We can maintain our favorite bread in our routine without worrying about high carbs. These pieces of bread will still have a simi-lar taste and texture the same way we love and like. Let's first have a look at some of the reasons why traditional bread tends to have high carbs. That is, the carbohydrates present in bread are starch and fiber. A lot of carbs can also invite health issues to our bodies. Firstly, most of the carbs come from substances such as fiber, which is a carb that cannot be digested and starch, this is a digestible form of carb.

In our case, we type of carbs we are supposed to avoid are the digestible types. This is because indigestible carbs are safe and convenient for a well-being digestive system. The digestible carbs are the ones that are converted to energy. When one hap-pens to take them more than they are required, the body stores it as fat. When digestible carbs are taken in this way, they will cause a gain in weight and lead to several health issues. So, with this in mind, we have to reduce our intake of the digestible form of carbs and change our diet to low carb. Baking wheat made from wheat is the contributor of carbs in the traditional bread. We can switch the flour that we use to bake low carb pieces of bread. The breads can be very similar to our favorite breads. When we avoid carbs, we tend to stabilize our blood pressure.

In this chapter, we will take an in-depth look at the different ideas on bread that we can use to reduce our weight. Let's first focus on people who want bread that is low in carbs. These are mostly people who are in a low carb diet. One of the pieces of bread that are low in carbs and is highly recommended for people in the diet is the cloud bread. Cloud bread is a big deal in weight loss practice. This bread has been gaining popular-ity since its conception. Apart from it being carb-free, it is also grain-free. Let us see how right this kind of bread can be to your health. It contains almost half of the calories in an ordinary bread.

Cloud bread is one of the leading foods in the world of healthy foods. Many people consider it to be from a fairy tale, but it is real and highly helpful. Cloud bread stand out from other traditional breads. It stands out because it contains a huge percentage of proteins that are very vital to the human body and overall wellbeing. The proteins present in a cloud bread are almost two grams in every cloud. This bread consists of very few ingredients. This fact makes it very easy to bake at home. The only disadvantage with a cloud bread is that it lacks fiber. Fiber has been proven to control cholesterol. Cloud bread I gluten-free. Gluten is a collective term referring to many different types of proteins. This is found in barley, triticale or rye.

Another fact about cloud bread is that it contains no carbs. People who are in a low carb diet should be thankful because their prayers have been answered. How are their prayers answered? This is because they seek bread that has no carbs, and cloud bread meets all their demands. This type of bread is carb-free, and it also has other health benefits. It is made mostly from cream bread that is cottage cheese. It has a straightforward recipe. If we change our perspective and focus on the micronutrients of the cloud bread, we find that it does not only contain proteins. It also contains vitamins A and D. It also contains mineral salts phosphorus, selenium, and choline. Most of these nutrients enhance human metabolism and optimum functioning. Another advantage that a cloud bread possesses is that, like an ordinary, it can also be frozen. It can also be prepared as a toast. To the foodies who like exploring new things, we can also use some spices in the recipe for making any cloud bread. Let us look at how we can create this carb-free delicacy.

The process involved in preparing cloud bread is not time-consuming. Since this type of bread is very delicate, it is supposed to be baked at allow temperature. This can increase the time of preparation, but we do this to avoid burning the bread in the process. The temperature that gives us the best of cloud bread is 300° Fahrenheit. Below is the ingredient list of cloud bread, these are the only ones required to make a keto bread;

> ➤ Eggs -These are the main component of the bread.
> ➤ Cream of tartar -This is required to stabilize the egg whites while whipping them.
> ➤ Greek yogurt -This adds the texture and some flavor. One can also use sour cream if he or she does not have Greek yogurt.
> ➤ Salt -This creates the main flavor of the bread.

It is a lot of fun to make cloud bread. Now let us look at how we can combine these ingredients to come up with the best cloud bread. First, we start with the eggs; place all the whites of our eggs on a big open bowl. After placing the eggs, we add the cream of tartar and whip the combination. If you do not have whipped these ingredients properly, the bread won't turn out the way it is supposed to turn out. We shall then add the Greek yogurt and salt while whipping till we obtain a smooth mixture.

In this step, we are going to fold the egg whites into the egg yolks until they combine. This should be done carefully so that we do not deflate the air in the eggs. Once all the ingredients are fully incorporated, the batter should thick. Then we are to mound the half of a cup of the batter onto a sheet lined together with a silicone mat. We can also use parchment paper instead of the silicone mat. Then we shape the mounds into half of the inch-thick disks. To form the cloud bread, we can use a spatula. Bake the bread for thirty minutes until it is dry to touch. The similarity between ordinary bread and cloud bread is the texture.

Cloud bread tastes mostly like eggs. This is because the main ingredient is eggs. This egg flavor tends to reduce as time goes by after baking the bread. Before using the bread, we are supposed to leave for an hour before we can use it. Just after baking, we store cloud bread in an airtight container. The texture of our cloud bread also reduces with time. This airtight container can be stored in a refrigerator. With our cloud bread stored in an airtight container, we can keep it up to three days at any room temperature, and it can survive for seven days when it is in a refrigerator.

There are different types of bread that are carb-free. We have already seen one of these types of bread. The second other bread is the almond flour keto bread. Let us look at how the almond flour is made first. Almonds are one of the oldest cultivated types of foods in the history of humankind. It is also named in the Old Testament. The Middle East is the origin of this important kind of plant. It came from countries like Turkey and Syria. With time it was spread into Africa and some European countries. Almond meals and almond flour are both from the same source that is ground almonds. The difference between the two have is the size of the individual grain.

Almond flour is the finest when the two are compared. Almonds were introduced into Europe as a form of a cookie. This cookie was known as maccherone. This type of cookie was introduced by the Sicilians. These cookies will be later dispersed to the next country, Italy. They were passed to France through Catherine de Medici. This spread happened in the 16th century. These cookies have now evolved to what we now call macaroons. They will take three hundred years in order to reach England. Due to the demand of low-carbs in recent years, Almond has once again gained its popularity. The almond flour tastes the same as the almond in its raw form. The almond flour has a lot of health benefits to the human body. Almond contains vitamins which are vital for the human to survive. The vitamins contained in almond are E, and multiple vitamin B. Vitamin B is essential in the growth of hair and normal nerve function. Almond also contains mineral salts that are important to the human body.

The minerals include manganese, calcium, and magnesium. They are available in large amounts in almonds. The human body needs manganese in small amounts to function normally. One of the purposes of manganese to the body is that it is a strong and efficient antioxidant. The most and important of all Almond advantages is it can assist with obesity. Almonds can play a huge role in weight loss. This is because it lacks fiber. As we know, fiber can make an individual feel fuller hence leading to a reduction in food intake. To get most of the nutrients from almonds, we need to ground up the almonds themselves. Another advantage is that it is also gluten-free. This means that it does not contain proteins that are related to any form of gluten.

Almond flour does not contain carbohydrates. So, this makes it the perfect flour in preparing bread for low carb diet people. This type of bread is low in carbs just as the flour used in making that particular type of bread. Research has shown that almonds can be compared to a big powerhouse in terms of health benefits. When it comes to losing weight, almonds contain very much complex carbohydrates that can assist in weight loss and maintaining a slimmer waistline.

According to research done by IJORMD on the effects of almond to people who were trying to lose weight. The people under study were given the same amount of proteins and the same number of calories each day. One-half of the people were given a low-calorie menu and also some mass of almonds each day. When had finished the study, the researchers noticed that half of the population that was given almonds as part of their diet had a more than fifty percent greater weight reduction. They also have a fifty percent reduction in their waist circumference. They also had a greater percentage of fat mass loss compared to the people who were not getting any almonds per day.

The research also shows that a low-calorie diet combined with almonds can and will improve one's health. So far, we have seen all the about how almond flour can be used to reduce weight. We are going to look at how we can convert all those advantages into a low carb bread for us to consume. If you are a beginner in low carb baking, no need to worry. We will go through on step by step in simple terms for you to understand what is going on and how to do it on your own practice.

Using almond flour to bake a low carb bread is simple to everyone despite their experience. Note that since almond flour does not contain gluten, the bread does not become soft and stretchy after baking. To make our bread soft and stretchy, we are going to use eggs for that purpose. We can also use psyllium, which absorbs water several times of its volume. This assists us in getting the structure and the volume we need in our low carb bread. This also results in the bread having more fiber. In order to bake an Almond bread, we need an oven heated to 350° Fahrenheit. We also need, of course, almond flour to prepare our delicacy. In our case, we shall be using Psyllium husk powder that is a quarter of a cup for an entire loaf. We can even use just two to three tablespoons for a whole bread. If we do this, we are supposed to reduce the amount of water we are going to use.

Our recipe requires minimal ingredients. The following is a perfect recipe for a keto almond flour bread. We are going to require the following ingredients. The first thing we take two eggs. Crack the two eggs into a bowl, and then we add two egg whites. This recipe gives its best when the eggs we are using are always at room temperature. Then we whisk the eggs for some time until they are frothy. The left-over egg yolks can be used to make home-based mayonnaise. Then we add psyllium husks with almond flour. After that, we introduce baking powder, water, salt, melted butter, and xanthan gum. Note that if you don't have xanthan gum, you are advised to use a lot of baking powder. Mix the ingredients until we have a smooth dough.

Finally, take the dough and put it in a loaf tin, if you have silicone loaf pan you are advised to use it. Smooth the topmost part of the dough. Do not press down on the dough. It is because we require as much air in the dough as possible. Bake for forty-five minutes. To determine if our bread is ready, insert a knife until it comes out clean.

A paleo diet can be compared to the hunter and gatherer diet of our human ancestors. It is not possible to determine which type of food they ate, but most researchers believe that they ate mostly whole foods. By having such a diet and having an active life, they had fewer cases of obesity and other related health issues. Many studies done show that this kind of diet can lead to a big and yet significant loss of body weight. In most cases, we cannot say there is a right way to eat.

So, a paleo diet is a diet that includes mostly whole foods. When a person is in a paleo diet, there are specific types of food and ingredients one has to avoid. These are grains, sugar, and high fructose corn syrup, legumes, and dairy. The simple law is if it is something from the factory, don't try and get it into your mouth. This is what is meant by the paleo diet. Coconut flour can be a perfect replacement for wheat flour. It is one of the most popular flour for low carb diet enthusiasts. It also has a little amount of gluten.

Coconut flour has an impressive nutrition profile. It can also offer other benefits. These benefits include blood pressure stability and can help in weight loss. In this section, we are going to look at how we can prepare coconut flour. Then use it for baking our low carb and nutritious bread for people who are in a low carb diet. To make the coconut flour, we have to dry the coconut flesh, and then we have to grind it to form a flour.

During this process, we first have to crack open the coconuts and drain the liquid that is present in it. We then scrap the coconut meat out, rinse it, then we grate it, and we finally strain it to separate the solid part from the milk. After doing this, the meat is baked in a low-temperature oven until it is scorched. What then follows is the dry meat being passed to a miller where it is ground into flour. One Property that makes coconut floor precious is that it is gluten-free. Let us look at the nutrients and beneficial facts of using coconut flour. What we are going to focus on is the use of coconut flour in the baking paleo coconut flour bread. Coconut flour may assist in shedding off excess weight.

The components that are present in coconut flour are fiber and protein. These two elements tend to reduce hunger and food appetite. Coconut also has MCTs, and these compounds are not likely to be stored in the human body as fat. The reason why these compounds are not stored as fat is that they are converted directly in the liver, and they are utilized to produce energy in the mitochondrion. MCTs can also reduce the appetite of an individual person greatly. They are also processed differently than the longer chain fats that are in nuts by the human body. This process accelerates the burning of calories in your body. However, such an event has very little effect. In recent studies, research has shown that using MCTs in place of long-chain fat helps people who are struggling with weight loss.

Let us now look at how we can prepare our low carb coconut flour bread at the comfort of our home. First, we will look at the ingredients that we require to bake this paleo coconut flour bread. This bread is mostly covered with seed. This keto paleo bread that is as a result of coconut flour is the perfect choice for a sandwich. This recipe also solves the problem of people who have nut allergies. This means that people who have nut allergies can have a taste of this bread. You will also notice that the ingredients we are going to use are most likely to be found in your kitchen. This bread is fluffy and also sliceable. We will be using at least one hour and around thirty minutes. Our bread will be sliced into seventeen slices. We are going to need an oven heated to 180° Celsius. Our ingredients are as follows;

- 10 Large eggs -We can use chicken eggs.
- ¾ cup of coconut flour.
- ¾ cup of butter.
- ½ teaspoon salt.
- ½ teaspoon of baking powder.
- ¾ teaspoon xanthan gum -This is just optional.

After heating the oven to the required temperature. You crack the eggs into the bowl and whip for at least a minute until the eggs are well combined. Take your coconut flour, baking flour, xanthan gum, salt, butter, and baking powder whip until they are entirely and thoroughly combined. This mixture should be a little bit thick. Place a parchment paper on a loaf tin then introduce the batter into the tin. Make sure the top of the batter is uniform. Bake for fifty minutes, to ensure the bread is ready a skewer should come out of the bread clean. To store our bread, we have to slice it before we preserve it in a fridge or freezer.

The next keto bread we will be looking at is the macadamia nut bread. This is made up of macadamia nuts. In the universe of nuts, it can be directly compared to gold because of its precious value. This exotic nut is very rich of its kind of flavor, and they can be served as dessert nuts. They are also offered as gifts during holiday times. The British colonists discovered these nuts while they were in Queensland, Australia. These nuts are a great source of iron, vitamin B, phosphorus, and calcium. In our lives, it's very hard to kick bread out of our menu. It is as if it was created so that we get hooked up to this stuff. This can be bad news for people who want to lose weight. The ultimate answer lies in the macadamia nut keto bread. Despite macadamia being a nut, it can be used to bake a low carb bread. Let's look at what we require to prepare this low carb macadamia nut bread. The ingredients are as follows;

- ➤ FBOMB macadamia pecan nut butter.
- ➤ Butter.
- ➤ Some eggs
- ➤ A little of almond flour.
- ➤ Baking powder.
- ➤ Salt.
- ➤ Xanthan gum.

First, we heat the oven to 350°. Use a greased parchment paper to line a loaf pan. Crack the eggs into a bowl and whip with an electric mixer. This whipping should at least take 2 -3 minutes. Use another bowl to mix all the other dry ingredients. Reduce the velocity of the mixer to low then the dry ingredients into the bowl with the wet ingredients. Once the ingredients are in one bowl, you can use a spoon to finish the mixing. Note that you have not supposed to mix the elements. Remove the butter from the bowl and transfer it to the loaf pan that you prepared in the beginning. Bake in the oven for 45 minutes. The bread should have little cracks at the top and golden brown in color. After baking leaves the bread for five minutes before serving the delicacy.

Let us look at the last keto bread that we are going to discuss. Garlic is a cousin to the ordinary onion that we use in the kitchen. It is a small but a goliath in the link at how it helps in weight loss. Garlic promotes weight loss by increasing the rate at which our bodies burn fat. A study done by researchers shows that aged garlic can lead to weight loss in specific women. The best thing from the research we now know that foods that burn fats are more efficient when used together with a little bit of garlic as an additive. Garlic also has an extra advantage; it adds taste to different kinds of food without adding any number of calories to the menu. Most people who use garlic as a remedy in weight loss continue using garlic since without garlic will lose its taste. Note that for better consumption of garlic, we have to cook it a little bit. The following are the ingredients that we require for our keto garlic bread.

- 1 c. shredded mozzarella.
- ½ c almond flour.
- 2 tablespoons cream cheese.
- 1 tablespoon garlic powder.
- 1 tablespoon baking powder.
- Kosher salt'.
- 1 large egg.
- 1 tablespoon butter that is melted.

- 1 clove garlic, this clove garlic should be minced.
- 1 tablespoon of fresh parsley that is chopped.
- 1 tablespoon of Parmesan.
- Marinara heated lightly for serving.

Before we proceed, we need to heat the oven to 400° Celsius. You are supposed to line a big baking sheet with parchment paper. Fist put the almond flour, mozzarella, cream cheese, garlic powder, and some of the salt into a bowl. Using a microwave, heat the butter until all the cheese melts. After heating the cheese, crack the egg. After combining all the ingredients, mix until you obtain a dough. Shape the dough into a ½ inch thick in the shape of an oval on your lined baking sheet that you prepared earlier. In another smaller bowl, take the garlic parmesan and parsley and mix them thoroughly. Take this mixture and using a brush, apply it on the top of the bread. Bake the dough until it is golden brown. This can take up to 17 minutes. When the bread is ready, it can be served with the marinara sauce.

References

FatForWeightLoss. (2019, September 6). Keto Bread [Blog post]. Retrieved from https://www.fatforweightloss.com.au/keto-bread/

Suazo, A. (n.d.). 30 Best Keto Bread Recipes That'll Make You Forget Carbs [Blog post]. Retrieved from https://www.bulletproof.com/recipes/keto-recipes/best-keto-bread-recipes-2g3c/

CHAPTER 4: SWEET AND SAVORY RECIPES

PEANUT BUTTER KETO COOKIE RECIPE

Compared to other homemade cookies, these keto-friendly cookies are by far very delicious and easy to prepare, as I will show you below. My recipe will yield 22 cookies and will take roughly between 1 hour and 2 hours from preparation to serving.

Ingredients

> One and a half cups of smooth melted unflavored peanut butter.
> One cup of coconut flour.
> 1/4 cup for packed of brown sugar, i.e., Swerve(Keto-Friendly).
> Coconut oil {1 tsp.}
> Kosher salt just one pinch
> Use chocolate chips which are dark, melted and keto-friendly {2 cups only}
> One tablespoon of unsweetened vanilla extract.

Directions

i) Start by making a smoothie paste using salt, an extract of vanilla, peanut butter, and even coconut flour.

ii) Prepare a baking sheet using baking paper. Use a small Oxo scoop, mold the mixture into small rounds and push them downwards slightly so that they are a bit flat on top and place them. You can freeze them so that they become firm. This might take one hour.

iii) Then you can mix the melted paste of chocolate with coconut oil and stir them thoroughly.

iv) You can coat the butter rounds using the melted paste. Solidifies the chocolate by adding more peanut butter.

This will take about ten minutes.

v)   Serve the cookie when cold. The leftovers can be stored in the freezer.

Nutritional facts based on one serving

Calories   73 g

Total fat   6.1g

Cholesterol   0g

Sodium   57.2mg

Potassium   0.3 g

Carbohydrates 3.7g

Protein   2.7g

AVOCADO BROWNIES

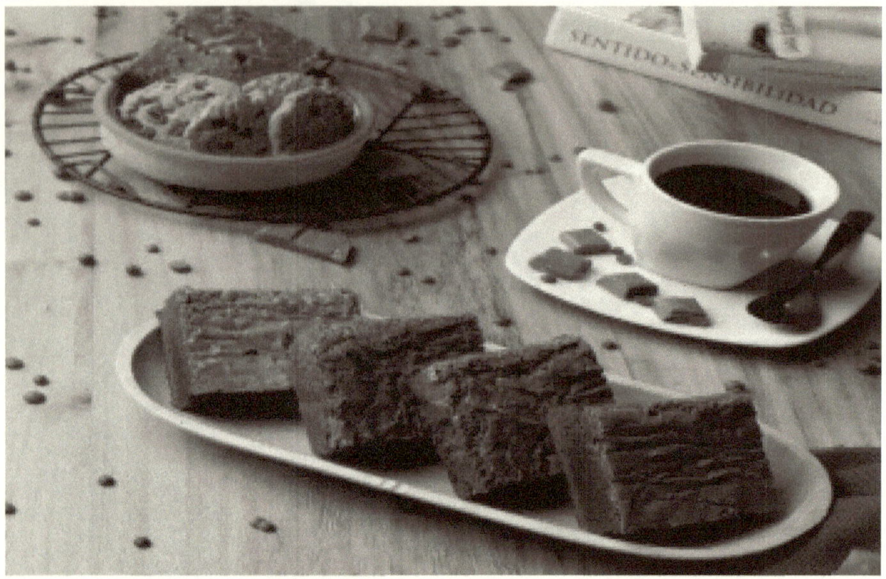

Have you been wondering how to make a keto-friendly dessert recipe? Avocado brownies are the best you will ever make. With their saccharine chocolate flavor and fudgy texture, you will love this gluten-free, low carb recipe. The total time required to prepare and serve is between 30 to 40 minutes.

Ingredients

- ➢ Ninety grams of natural dark chocolate.
- ➢ 2 tsp of coconut oil.
- ➢ I cup of ripened avocado paste.

- Two eggs.
- ½ cup keto friendly crystal sweetener. i.e., a mixture of Stevia and Erythritol sweeteners.
- 70 grams of almond meal.
- ½ cup unflavored cocoa powder
- ½ tsp(teaspoon) baking soda
- ¼ tsp teaspoon salt
- 1 tsp vanilla extract
- Glazing Ingredients
- ¼ tsp coconut virgin oil
- 12 g crushed and salted roast pecan nuts
- 40 g keto melted chocolate bites
- 1 tablespoon of sea salt

Instructions:

1. The oven should be preheated to 180 Celsius.
2. Line a pan, preferably a square brownie with baking paper.
3. Put the oil and chocolate bites in a saucepan and heat until all the chocolate melts. Alternatively, you can heat both ingredients in a microwave until the chocolate melts.
4. In a food processor with a Sabatier blade, put all the ingredients except for the glazing ingredients. That is the avocado flesh, erythritol, eggs, almonds, melted chocolate, an extract of vanilla, coco powder, baking powder, baking soda, and even salt.
5. Stir until all the ingredients mix and form a thick brownie batter.
6. Put the brownie mixture in the ready saucepan and slather evenly using a spatula.
7. Bake the brownie for thirty minutes. To know if it is ready, insert a skewer into the brownie. If it comes out untainted, the brownie is ready.
8. Let the brownie cool for ten minutes so that you

can pull it out easily from the pan by the baking paper.

9. Switch the brownie to a cookie rack and cool it down to room temperature.

10. For the chocolate glazings, heat the chocolate bits, and coconut oil under medium heat until the chocolate melts.

11. Sprinkle the melted chocolate bites on the brownie. You can opt to decorate the brownie by drizzling the pecan nuts along with the sea salt on the brownie.

12. Divide the brownie into 16 square pieces and put them in the pantry in a sealed container for at least four days.

Key takeaway:

Net carbs in a slice of brownie slice amount to 3.5g

Other nutritional information based on one serving

Nutrition Facts per slice of brownie

2.4 grams -------------------- proteins

2.4 grams ----------------- sugar

225kcal -------------------- calories

2.5 grams------------------- fiber

6 grams-------------------carbohydrates

6.4 grams----------------- fat

EGG MUFFINS WITH VEGGIES AND SAUSAGES

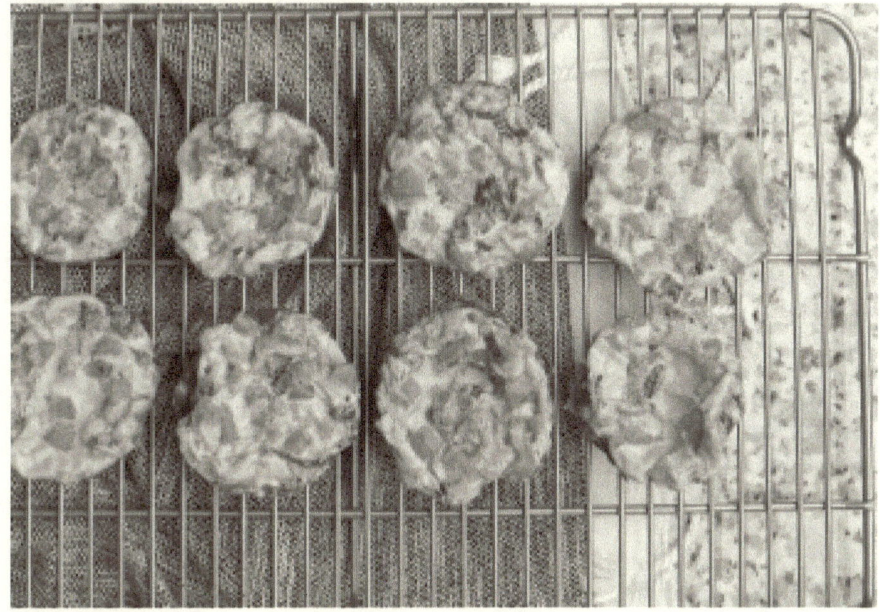

Ingredients

- ➤ Six large eggs
- ➤ Ground sausage
- ➤ ½ cup red diced onions
- ➤ ½ teaspoon of Salt
- ➤ ¼ teaspoon of thyme (dried)
- ➤ ¼ cup of chopped Basil
- ➤ ½ cup of cheese, preferably parmesan.
- ➤ 1/2 cup diced bell peppers
- ➤ ½ cup chopped broccoli florets

Method

1. Heat the oven to 162 Celsius.
2. Beat the eggs together. Add Basil, pepper, salt,

thyme, and stir.

3. In a medium-sized pan, heat the sausage. Once it turns brown, add the vegetables and cook for approximately ten minutes until they turn tender.
4. Add parsley and fresh Basil and stir.
5. Spray non-stick cooking oil to a twelve-cup muffin medium-sized pan.
6. Put a 1 ½ tablespoon and ½ of the blended meat into the cup and add one tablespoon of cheese to the mixture.
7. Add ¼ cup of beaten egg mixture to each cup and bake the mix for ten to 15 minutes.
8. Cool the egg muffins for about five minutes and remove them from the Pan cups.
9. You can also choose to drizzle parsley and Basil on the muffins for tastier muffins before serving.

Nutritional facts based on one serving

Calories	124kcal
Total fat	9g
Cholesterol	102mg
Sodium	321mg
Potassium	132mg
Carbohydrates	2g
Protein	7g
Vitamins	12.9%
Calcium	78%
Iron	0.8%
Saturated fat	3g

Vitamin A   485%

KETO SNICKERDOODLES

Requirements:

- ¼ teaspoon of kosher salt
- Refined almond flour {2 cups}
- 3/4 cup erythritol powdered sweetener
- 1/2 teaspoon of baking soda
- Softened salted butter {1/2 cup}
- One teaspoon of mashed cinnamon

Method

1. Heat the pan beforehand to about 350 degrees Fahrenheit.
2. Mix the almond flour, softened salted butter, kosher salt, and the sweetener to a stiff dough in a large bowl.
3. Roll the stiff dough into sixteen equal balls.
4. Whisk the sweetener and cinnamon together in a medium-sized dish.
5. Roll the small balls into the cinnamon mixture and coat evenly.
6. Line a parchment cookie sheet and spread slightly.
7. You can take about 14 minutes to bake it.
8. Let them cool and serve.

Nutritional facts based on one serving

Calories	135 g
Total fat	12g
Cholesterol	0g
Sugars	1g

Total Carbohydrates   5g

Net Carbohydrates   2g

Protein   3g

CHOCOLATE CHIP COOKIE ICE CREAM

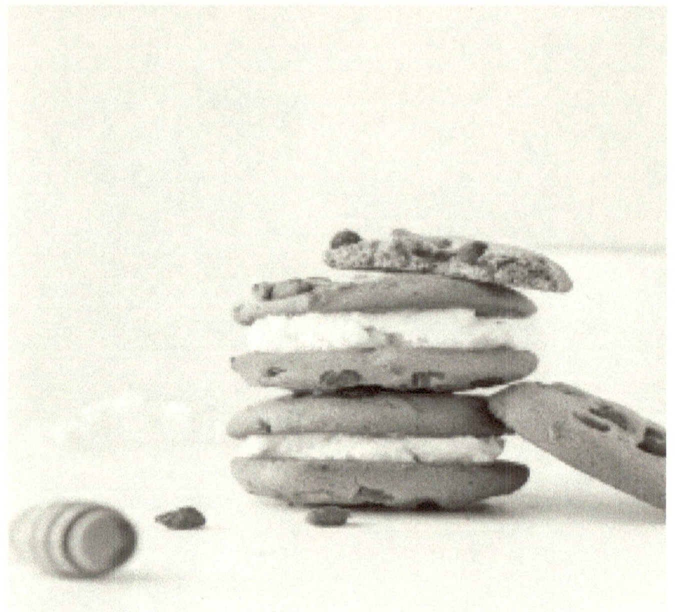

Preparation time to serving takes between 10 minutes and 35 minutes.

Ingredients

- 500 g of thick whipping cream.
- ½ cup ground erythritol/ stevia blend
- Two teaspoons of unsweetened Vanilla extract
- One teaspoon of unsweetened peppermint extract
- 1 cup of almond milk(unsweetened)
- Eighty-five grams chopped of stevia flavored chocolate.

Method

1. Put the whipped cream into a large bowl. Using a

cream whipper, beat the cream until it gets stiff and peaked.
2. Add the sweetener in small proportions, stirring the mixture after each addition.
3. Whisk the peppermint and vanilla extracts in a medium-sized bowl.
4. Add the unsweetened milk in small proportions as you stir.
5. Store the mixture in a freezer. Afterward, add the chocolate bars and whisk them in.
6. Move the mixture to an airtight container and back to the freezer. This will make the ice cream to harden more before serving.

Nutritional facts based on one serving

Calories	255 g
Total fat	26g
Sugars	1g
Total Carbohydrates	6g
Fiber	3g
Protein	2g

KETO-FRIENDLY PEPPERONI PIZZA

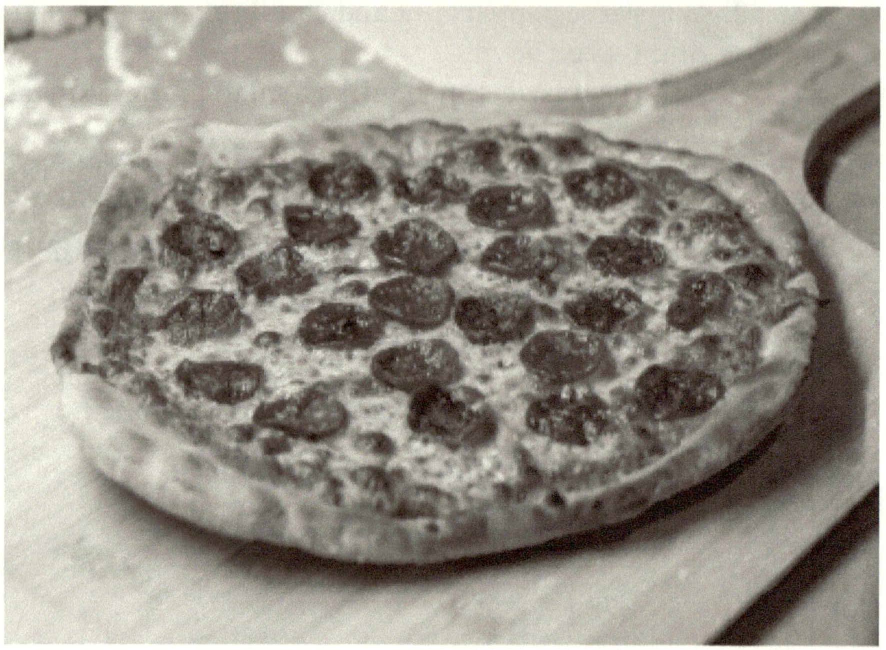

Ingredients

- ➢ 2 tsp. of yeast
- ➢ ½ cup of warm water
- ➢ 3 cups skim mozzarella cheese (shredded part)
- ➢ One egg(beaten)
- ➢ 1 cup ground almond flour
- ➢ One tsp. xanthan gum
- ➢ A pinch of salt
- ➢ Sliced pepperoni (2 ounces)
- ➢ ¼ cup sugar-free pizza sauce
- ➢ 1 optional ripe pepper flakes

The total cook time from preparation to serving takes about 35 minutes.

Method

1. Heat the oven to 190 degrees Celsius and prepare the baking sheet using parchment paper.
2. Add the warm water into the yeast and stir to dissolve.
3. In a medium-sized microwave bowl, put the mozzarella cheese and cover. Heat in the microwave for 1 minute 30 seconds until it melts completely. Add the yeast mixture plus the egg and whisk together. At this point, the mixture is not well mixed.
4. Add the xanthan gum, almond flour, and salt. If unable to properly mix, heat the cheese again in the microwave if necessary, to make the cheese soft. Whisk together until the mixture incorporates fully. Using your hands, knead the dough for 3 minutes.
5. Place the kneaded dough on the parchment baking paper and using your fingers, press into the dough to form a thin crust a few inches in diameter.
6. Bake the dough in the oven until it turns brown for about 11 minutes. Sprinkle pizza sauce on the pizza and top it using the mozzarella cheese. Don't forget to spread pepperoni on the pizza as a top-up as well.
7. Return the pizza to the oven to bake again for about 6 minutes, which gives the cheese enough time to melt.
8. Additionally, you can also spread the red pepper flakes on to the pizza.
9. Cut the pizza into slices and serve.

Nutrition facts

Nutritional facts based on one serving

Calories   336 kcal

Total fat	24.3 g
Cholesterol	77mg
Sodium	639mg
Total Carbohydrates	8.5g
Protein	22g

CHOCOLATE PEANUT BUTTER POPSICLES

These nutty spread popsicles are a definitive low carb choice for peanut butter enthusiasts. These sugar-free ice pops dunked in dim make for a tasty keto treat. If you are as entirely a bit of a chocolate fan and peanut butter as I am, you definitely know these are great, yet I will underline that point in any case. They are truly great, and each individual from my family unit was a big fan.

Ingredients

- ➤ Softened cream cheese (7 oz.)
- ➤ 1/2 cup ground Swerve Sweetener
- ➤ 1/2 teaspoon vanilla concentrate
- ➤ 3 1/4 cup substantial cream
- ➤ 4 ounces of sugar-free chopped chocolate bars
- ➤ 1/2 ounce chopped cocoa butter
- ➤ Unsweetened and creamy peanut butter {1 cup}

Method

1. In a huge bowl, whisk together the vanilla concentrate, sweetener, cream cheese, the heavy cream, and the peanut butter until a smooth paste is formed.
2. Add 12 to 15 spoons of Popsicle molds (contingent upon size) and tap the molds solidly on the counter to discharge all the trapped air bubbles.
3. Put Popsicle sticks in the focal point of each Popsicle mold (wooden sticks are best as they remain in the popsicles longer without dislodging).
4. Freeze the popsicles for 4 hours until they are firm. Remove the popsicle sticks from the molds by run-

ning the molds under hot boiled water, then delicately contort the sticks until they discharge from
the molds. Keep the molds in a cooler until you get
to dip the chocolate.

5. Line a parchment baking sheet in the cooler and
   leave it spread.
6. Place a metal bowl indirectly over a pan of hot
   water (don't let the pot get into contact with the
   water).
7. Add the cocoa butter and ground chocolate to the
   bowl and whisk together until all the chocolate
   is liquefied. Remove the pot from heat and set it
   aside.
8. Dip a popsicle halfway into the chocolate paste,
   and let the excess trickle off into the bowl (Twist
   the popsicle around while the chocolate drips to
   get even more exciting chocolate drips).
9. At the point when the chocolate solidifies around
   the popsicle, place the completed popsicle on the
   baking sheet inside the cooler.
10. Repeat steps 8 and 9 for all the remaining pop-
    sicles.

Nutrition facts

Nutritional facts based on one serving (1 Popsicle)

Calories   280 kcal

Total fat   24.9 g

Fiber   5.6g

Total Carbohydrates 8.7g

Protein   5.6g

KETO CHICKEN ENCHILADA BOWL

This Mexican dish is easy to make and happens to have a shallow carb concentration. It is incredibly yummy and filling. Below, I am going to show you how I made a Keto Chicken Enchilada Bowl dish on a stovetop. Yet, it can be made without much of a stretch on an instant Pot by cooking the chicken, chills, onions and enchilada sauce together on low heat throughout the day.

You can also prepare the chicken sauce mixture early and freeze it for later use. When you need it, allow it to defrost and heat it on the stovetop. Then, add fresh toppings and cauliflower rice to complete the dish.

Another alternative is to prepare the cauliflower individually. In case you are still curious about the dish, it's quite straightforward. Just ground the cauliflower that you can set yourself up using a food processor and a new cauliflower head. The best approach, however, to prepare this delicious meal is described below.

Ingredients

- ➤ 1 Tomato
- ➤ ½ cup sour cream
- ➤ 1 1/2 tablespoon of coconut oil
- ➤ ¼ cup chopped pickled jalapenos
- ➤ 1 cup sliced cheddar cheese
- ➤ One avocado
- ➤ ½ cup sour cream
- ➤ Two chopped onions
- ➤ ¾ cups of enchilada sauce
- ➤ 0.25 ml cup of water
- ➤ One skinless and Boneless chicken thigh

➤ One 500g can of green chills

Method

Melt the coconut oil over medium heat using either a Dutch oven or any other desired non-stick cooking pot. When hot, burn chicken thighs until gently darker.

Add in the enchilada sauce and a cup of water, then add the green chilies and onions and stir.

Reduce heat to medium heat and cover the pot. Let the chicken cook for 30 minutes until the chicken becomes tender and is thoroughly cooked.

Transfer the chicken to a kitchen table and mince the chicken to smaller pieces and return the chopped pieces into the cooking pot.

Bubble the chicken under small heat for an extra 12 minutes to allow the chicken to retain flavor and enable the sauce to come down a bit.

To serve, top with jalapeno, avocado, tomato, cheddar, and sour. You can tweak the toppings to your liking.

If you so wish, serve the chicken delicacy individually or with cauliflower rice.

Nutrition facts

Nutritional facts based on one serving (Keto Chicken Enchilada Bowl)

Calories	568 kcal
Total fat	40.21 g
Fiber	4.27g

Total Carbohydrates   6.14g

Protein   38.38g

LOW CARB TACO CABBAGE SKILLET

This Low Carb Taco Cabbage Skillet is a simple dinner recipe with an astonishing taco seasoning flavor.

When you don't have much time to cook a delicious, nutritious, and low carb dinner, then this recipe is the perfect choice for you. That is because to make it, you essentially toss everything into a cooking pan, and stir it until the meal is ready.

When you are busy with no opportunity to consider what you are going to cook, then you should find this simple, easy meal. What's more, if your family loves tacos, then they will most likely love this taco recipe. Make sure to make extra so that you can have remained for lunch tomorrow.

Ingredients

- 16 ounces of minced beef
- ½ cup of salsa
- 2 cups shredded cabbage
- Two teaspoons of chili powder
- Three ¼ cups of shredded cheese
- Pepper and salt
- Optional seasons
- Green onions
- Sour cream

Method

1. Cook the beef in a skillet until it turns brown and drains the fat
2. Add the seasoning, cabbage, and salsa to the cooking pan and boil mildly.
3. Cover and lower the heat and cook for 10 minutes

    until the cabbage turns soft.

4. Ultimately minimize the heat and add the cheese. stir until the cheese melts

5. Flavor the food to your liking with green onions, sour cream, avocado, or any other chosen toppings.

Nutrition facts

Nutritional facts based on one serving (Low Carb Taco Cabbage Skillet)

Calories	325 kcal
Total fat	21 g
Fiber	1g
Total Carbohydrates	5g
Net Carbohydrates	4g
Protein	30g

KETO DINNER ROLLS

This recipe is incredibly easy to make, totally heavenly, and remarkably filling. The filling effect is brought about by the additional flax seeds added to the recipe. The flax seeds are full of fiber and give the dinner rolls a full sweet flavor.

This is the perfect Keto bread formula I've at any point attempted, so I'm particularly glad to share it on the book. The rolls will most likely replace typical bread from your diet to add to your low carbohydrate diet.

These Keto supper rolls can be eaten without any other food combination or eaten in pizza crust form or as a hamburger bun.

Ingredients

- ➤ One cup of shredded mozzarella.
- ➤ 1-ounce cream cheese
- ➤ 1 cup almond flour
- ➤ ¼ cup crushed flax seeds
- ➤ One large egg
- ➤ ½ teaspoon of baking soda

Method

1. Preheat the stove to 401 degrees Celsius.
2. Line the baking sheet with parchment material and store it in a safe place.
3. In a medium-sized bowl, liquefy the mozzarella and cream cheddar together and microwave for 1 min.
4. Stir the cheeses together until they become smooth, add the egg and mix until they consolidate
5. In another bowl, combine ground flaxseed, almond flour, and baking soda.

6. Blend the cheddar and egg mixture until the dough forms a softball that is sticky to the fingers.
7. Roll the balls in sesame seeds and place them onto the prepared baking sheet
8. Bake the rolls for 12 minutes until they are brilliantly dark colored
9. Let them cool for 15 minutes.

Nutrition facts

Nutritional facts based on one serving (1 roll)

Calories	219 kcal
Total fat	18g
Fiber	3.3g
Total Carbohydrates	5.6g
Net Carbohydrates	2.3g
Protein	10.7g

Key Notes

Coconut flour is certifiably not an immediate substitute for almond flour, and you should modify the amount.

The dough should be clingy to the fingers yet ought to have the option to shape balls. Utilize wet hands to the balls. In the event that the dough is entirely too wet even to allow molding, at that point, include an extra tablespoon of almond flour until it becomes malleable.

Four huge ball rolls work incredible for burgers and sandwiches. For supper rolls, use six smaller balls. Rolls may appear to be delicately soft when leaving the oven. However, they solidify as they cool.

KETO WHITE CHICKEN CHILI

In case you are wondering how you can have a delicious chili meal without beans in the serving, then this recipe will show you how to. To top it up, you can go ahead and add vegetables and chicken to boost the flavor. The chili is custom made using spicy jack cheese, shredded chicken, and peppers. Though not as thick as the traditional chili, the filling effect of the chill is very impressive.

Ingredients

- 450 grams of chicken breast
- 1 ½ cups chicken soup
- Two minced garlic cloves
- 130 grams chopped green chills
- One jalapeno (diced)
- One green pepper(diced)
- 0.25 ml cup diced of onion.
- Four tablespoons butter
- 0.25 ml cup heavy whipped cream
- 113 gm cream cheese
- Two teaspoons cumin
- One teaspoon oregano
- 0.25 teaspoon (optional)cayenne
- Salt and pepper (for adding taste)

Method

1. In a large cooking pot, season the chicken breasts with cayenne, oregano, salt, cumin, and pepper.
2. Over medium heat, Char both sides of the breasts until they turn golden.
3. Add the chicken soup to the cooking pot and cover. Cook the chicken for 20 mins. until it is thoroughly cooked.
4. With the chicken still cooking in the pot, melt the butter in a medium-sized skillet.

5. Add diced jalapeno, chills, onions, and green pepper to the skillet and cook until the vegetables soften.
6. Add the garlic cloves and cook for an additional 40 seconds and turn off the heat.
7. The moment the chicken is thoroughly cooked, mince it to smaller pieces and add them to the chicken broth.
8. Add the cooked vegetables to mix with the broth and chicken, and bring to mild heat for 11 minutes
9. Place the cream cheese in a medium bowl and microwave for 20 seconds until you can stir the mixture.
10. Add the cream cheese mixture into the pot with the vegetables and chicken.
11. Cook on low heat for an extra 16 minutes.

Nutrition facts

Nutritional facts based on one serving (1 cup)

Calories	481 kcal
Total fat	30g
Fiber	1g
Total Carbohydrates	5g
Net Carbohydrates	4g
Protein	39g

KETO BROCCOLI CHEDDAR SOUP

The soup is incredibly filling and yummy. In addition, the soup is delicious, low carb, and very creamy.

The total time required to prepare the soup and serve is roughly about 20 minutes.

Ingredients

- Two tablespoons Butter.
- 1/8 cup white onion
- 0.5 teaspoon finely minced garlic
- 2 cups Chicken soup broth
- Pepper and salt, to taste
- 1 cup of chopped Broccoli
- One tablespoon keto cream cheese
- 0.25 ml cup Whipping cream(Heavy)
- 1 cup shredded Cheddar cheese
- Two slices crumbled and cooked Bacon.
- ½ tsp. Xanthan gum

Method

1. In a medium-sized pot, heat the butter until it melts. Add the garlic and onion and heat using medium heat to the point of the onions turn golden in color or become translucent and soft.
2. Add the broccoli and broth to the pot and stir. The broccoli should cook until it turns soft. Add pepper, salt, and any other seasoning ingredients of your choice.
3. Put the cheese in a bowl and heat in the microwave for 30 seconds until it turns soft and can easily be stirred.
4. Add the cream cheese and whipping cream into the

    soup and boil mildly.

5. Switch off the heat, add as soon as you do so, add and stir the cheese (cheddar).
6. If you so wish, you can add the xanthan gum and stir until the soup thickens.
7. Serve the soup when it is still hot alongside bacon crumbles.

Nutrition facts

Nutritional facts based on one serving (1 cup)

Calories	285 kcal
Total fat	24g
Fiber	1g
Total Carbohydrates	5g
Net Carbohydrates	2g
Protein	12g

CHAPTER 5: FAT BOMBS

Spicy Fat Bomb, Almond-Coconut, Cheese Fat Bombs in Bacon, Neapolitan, Almond Coconut

Fat bombs are low-carb vegan-friendly, Keto no-bake treats made with ingredients such as cream cheese, coconut oil, avocado, and butternut. What makes fat bombs healthy is the fact that they have little to no sugar. People suffering from diabetes find fat bombs a healthy option. You can include favorable ingredients to turn your fat bomb into a delicious treat. You need to choose your ingredients carefully if you want to make a delightful fat bomb. By now, you have seen trendy fat bombs on social media platforms. Many people search for recipes online in attempts to learn how to make fat bombs at home. A snack that is loved by many is freeze balls of coconut butter. Others prefer a mix of chia seeds, peanut butter, and cocoa powder. Fat bombs are great snacks for those who love rich desserts that are not too sweet.

Fat bombs can be eaten at any time because they are low in sugar. Some people think that such treats are reserved for people with health issues, but that is not the case. Fat bombs are not bland, and neither are they reserved for certain people. Incorporate fat bombs in your breakfast, post-workout snack, or a nighttime treat. People have different views regarding how much fat to eat in a day. The good thing with fat bombs is that they are high in hearty fat and free of refined sugar and carbohydrates. Moreover, you feel satiated fast because of the fat.

They are not candies or cookies which you eat plenty and still feel hungry. Despite their benefits, eat fat bombs with moderation. As it is said, too much of anything is dangerous. Fat bombs are treats made with almond, coconut oil, or cream cheese. People on keto diet love fat bombs because they are satisfying and tasty snacks that give healthy fats and little carbs. For the longest time, people thought that they needed lots of carbs to be satiated but is false. Keto diet has proven that you don't need to eat a bunch of carbs to be healthy or full. There are several keto fat bombs you can add to your diet.

You can indulge in decadent pecan pie fudge bombs at any time. This fat bomb is made with cacao butter, coconut butter, and pecans. To make this delicious treat, you will need ½ cup cacao butter, ½ cup coconut butter, 2 pieces of cacao, ½ chopped pecans, and 2tbps stevia. Start by adding pecans to a pot and toast for 5 minutes. Remove from the heat once it turns golden brown. Let it cool before chopping it up. Add the rest of the ingredients to a pan and melt on low heat. Add stevia and adjust according to desired taste. Remove from the heat and transfer to silicone molds. Put in the freezer for 2 hours. Serve.

You can also make keto mocha fat bombs to switch up your diet. If you are a fan of coffee, and nut butter, you will love mocha fat bombs. They melt in your mouth and boost your energy. For this recipe, you will need ½ cup keto butter, ¼ melted ghee, expresso, ¼ cup heavy cream, 1tbps vanilla extract, and a dash of salt. Blend all the ingredients in a food processor. Mix everything until smooth, and add sweetener to your liking. Pour to silicon molds, put in the freezer for 1 hour. Once it is firm, you can serve. Another great alternative is the Keto Butter Coconut Bites. It is made with nuts and is full of nutrients and low in sugar. The key ingredients are Keto chocolate collagen, coconut butter, nut butter, and coconut oil. Start by melting the coconut oil and mix it with the Keto Collagen in a bowl. Put the liquid in muffin tins and place in the freezer for 15 minutes. Remove from the freezer and spread softened coconut butter over it. Return the mixture to the freezer for another 15 minutes. Take from the freezer and spread Keto butter over it. Freeze for another hour. Serve.

Spicy fat bombs are convenient to have in hand to help you avoid eating unhealthy foods. Similar to many keto recipes, fat bombs are made with dark chocolate, peanut butter, or low glycemic sweeteners like stevia and syrup. Some people believe that fat bombs help in losing weight. Because fat bombs have 90 percent fat, they keep you in deep ketosis. Some people use fat bombs as snacks to maintain the ketogenic diet. Keeping ketosis requires you to take 70 percent of daily calories, which is difficult. Therefore, including fat bombs in your meals can help you consume your fat intake objective. Doing this will help you stay in ketosis and improve your weight loss journey. Below are fat bomb recipes you can make.

Ingredients

- ½ cup cacao butter
- 3 tsp almond butter
- 3 tsp peanut butter
- 3 tsp coconut butter
- ¼ monk fruit sweetener
- ¼ raw cacao powder

Instructions

1. Put a glass over a pot with simmering water and put coconut oil or cacao butter. Let it melt until it is liquid.
2. Add monk fruit, syrup or stevia, and cacao powder and stir until it is well mixed. Turn off the heat and stir the mixture until it cools down but remains liquid.

3. Put liquid chocolate in a silicone mold up to 2/3 and add ½ teaspoon coconut butter, ½ almond butter to the mixture. Pour chocolate on top and freeze for 30 minutes.
4. Take out the mold and serve.

It is important to know the nutritional information of the fat bombs. This one has 75 calories, and saturated fat contains 38% daily value. Fiber is 4%, protein 2%, sugar 1% and potassium 1%. The nutritional value of this fat bomb demonstrates that it is suitable for everyone. You don't have to worry about your calorie intake while taking this treat because it covers all your areas of concern.

You can also incorporate spicy fat bombs into your meals too. Pumpkin keto fat bombs have everything you need and are a great way to cure your sweet tooth. Moreover, spicy fat bombs allow you to hit your daily macros. The holidays are considered the hardest times to stick to healthy eating patterns, but the trick to staying on the course is a little indulgence. Spicy fat bombs are ideal for any occasion. They are meant to help you hit your macros and help the body burn fats. Each keto pumpkin spicy fat bomb has 1 carb, 0 protein, 4g fat, and 43 calories. You need to calculate the specific ingredients because macros vary depending on different brands.

Ingredients for spicy pumpkin fat bomb

1. ½ cup butter
2. 1 tablespoon pumpkin pie
3. ½ cup pumpkin
4. 2 packets stevia sweetener
5. 1/3 cup cream cheese
6. ½ tsp vanilla extract
7. ¼ teaspoon salt

Instructions

1. Add cream cheese and softened butter to a mixing bowl. Microwave the two for 20 seconds and stir to blend.
2. Add the remaining ingredients and stir to mix well
3. Use small cupcakes or pour into a mold
4. Freeze for 3-4 hours before serving
5. Keep in an airtight container, thaw a few minutes before serving.

Low-carb pumpkin spicy fat bombs are an easy and quick dessert treat recipe. Many people are afraid of trying the keto diet because they are afraid of giving up their favorite foods. They think that keto is boring and has no known benefits. However, this is far from the truth as keto has delicious treats like spicy fat bombs that make a difference to your meal. They transform your meal into a treat every time you incorporate them.

Keto pumpkin spicy fat bomb tips to keep in mind is that in other fat bomb recipes, a serving of oil is added, but should be avoided in this case because it weighs down the spice taste. Use two bombs as one serving to have desired results.

To make keto low-carb pumpkin spice fat bombs, you will need certain ingredients. This fat bomb is a quick dessert treat recipe that is perfect for ketosis lifestyles and diets. It tastes like pie and is gluten-free. Moreover, it is full of healthy fats and only has

1g of carbs. You need to prep the ingredients for 10 minutes, and the cooking time is 2 hours.

Ingredients

1. 1 tsp vanilla extract
2. 4 oz. cream cheese
3. 4 tsp melted butter
4. ½ cup pumpkin puree
5. 1 tsp ground cinnamon
6. 1 tsp chopped ginger
7. ½ nutmeg

Instructions

1. Put the ingredients to a bowl
2. Use a mixer to mix the ingredients for a few minutes until it is smooth
3. Line a mini cupcake pan with liners or not
4. Spoon the mixture into a muffin tin
5. Smooth the top of the fat bombs with a knife or spoon
6. Freeze for 2 hours
7. Serve

Notes

1. You can opt to buy pumpkin spice seasoning in place of listed above
2. In some fat bomb recipes, you can add coconut oil, but in this one, the taste of the oil overpowers the spicy taste
3. The spicy fat bombs melt if left at room temperature. To avoid this from happening, freeze all the remaining fat bombs immediately. Be on the lookout during the entire process.

Alternatively, you can make spiced cocoa coolers if you want to try something different. This fat bomb has 1.1g net carbs, 0.7g proteins, 5g fat, and 49kcal calories.

Ingredients

1. 1 tsp cinnamon
2. 2 tsp unsweetened cocoa powder
3. ¼ cayenne pepper
4. 15 drops of vanilla extract or stevia
5. 2 tsp swerve
6. Whipping cream

Instructions

1. Warm up the cream to help the ingredients dissolve easily
2. Mix ingredients with the cream
3. Pour out the mixture in an ice cube tray
4. Freeze for 2 hours
5. Serve

Notes

- Pick ingredients carefully
- Choose ingredients in their natural form

Net carbs	Protein	Fat	Calories
Coconut mil			
0.6 g	0.6 g	5.0 g	45 kcal
Cacao			
0.2 g	0.1 g	0.3 g	3 kcal
Vanilla extract	0 g	1 g	1 kcal
Cinnamon			
0.1 g	1 g	2g	1 kcal
Spices			

0 g	1 g	1g	2kcal
Erythritol			
0.2 g	1g	1 g	1 kcal
Stevia 1g	1 g	2 g	1 kcal
Total per serving, 2 pieces			
1.3 g	0.9 g	5 g	49 kcal

ALMOND COCONUT FAT BOMBS

Keto almond coconut fat bombs are amazing treats that everyone should taste. The good thing with them is that they take little time and effort to make. They are ideal for anyone on a ketogenic diet as they increase fat intake and keep carbs low. It is imperative to eat enough fat when on a ketogenic diet. Fat bombs are a great option to increase the amount of fat that you consume to help you reach ketosis faster. One keto fat bomb has 13.1g fat, 0.5g fiber, and 1.1g net carbs.

Ingredients for almond coconut fat bombs

- Coconut cream- coconut cream is the same as coconut milk. You can use coconut milk if you cannot find coconut cream.
- Almond butter- ensure that your almond butter has no added sugar. It is better to use smooth almond butter
- Erythritol- this is the best sweetener to use. It has no effect on your sugar levels and gives awesome sweetness. There are also other sweeteners that don't spike your sugar levels.
- Almonds- you can use almonds or macadamia nuts.
- Vanilla extracts- whip up vanilla extracts to use in this recipe and get all the juiciness.

Instructions

- Mix the almond coconut cream in a small bowl. Continue mixing until you get a smooth consistency. Add vanilla extract and the sweetener. Put the almond coconut cream in a freezer for 20- 30 minutes.
- Shape the balls. Remove the almond coconut from the fridge. It should be hard enough to form balls. Use a tablespoon scoop to form the balls. In the almond coconut is runny, put back to the freeze and let it sit for 20 minutes. You can add a thickener to it. Press the macadamia nut into the balls and add shredded coconut to them. You can roll the almond coconut balls in the shredded coconut.
- Put the almond coconut balls back to the freeze and allow them to sit for 1 hour.
- Serve and enjoy

Coconut almond fat bombs are delicious treats that can be enjoyed anytime. They are healthy, vegan, and low in carbs, which makes them perfect for staying in ketosis.

Nutrition Information

Servings **6**

The number of calories in the serving is 134, and the total fat is 21%. Protein consists of 5%, fiber 2%, and carbs 1%.

You can increase your intake of healthy fats easily without adding carbs. You can eat low carb desserts with the same macro as the fat fast recipe. If you don't have the time to prepare meals, this recipe is perfect for you. It takes less time and tastes good every time.

ALMOND COCONUT FAT BOMB INGREDIENTS

Crust

- Dash salt
- 3 oz. macadamia nuts
- 4tbps almond butter
- 6tbsp melted coconut oil
- ¼ cup shredded coconut

Chocolate layer

- ➤ 2 tbsp. coconut oil
- ➤ Stevia
- ➤ 6tbps cocoa powder

Coconut layer

- ✓ ¼ cup of shredded coconut
- ✓ 6tbsp melted coconut oil

Directions

1. Start by making the crust layer. Crush the salt macadamia nuts until finely ground. Put in almond butter and mix well. Put the mixture in a pan.
2. Make the coconut layer by mixing shredded coconut and coconut oil. When it is mixed well, spread it on top of the crush and put it aside.
3. Make the chocolate layer by mixing the coconut oil and cocoa powder and put drops of a sweetener of choice. Pour the mixture over the coconut layer and smooth it with a spatula. Put in the freezer for

2 hours.
4. Check from time to time to check whether it is ready.
5. Remove from the freezer after 2 hours and serve.

CHEESE FAT BOMBS IN BACON

Having a sweet tooth is a significant weakness in the keto diet because other times, you need long for sweet food. It can be frustrating if you long for sweet treats but have no access to it. Just because it is sweet, it does mean that it must be healthy. What most people have not realized is that you can enjoy a cheese fat bomb in bacon and get the same taste your favorite meals. In fact, when you taste a cheese fat bomb, you will have no interest in other treats. People on keto diet love incorporating fat cheese bombs in bacon because it is a nice way to enjoy a tasty meal. They would rather give up their bread, or rice and get the fat bomb dessert. That is how much people are serious about their fat cheese bombs. Cheesecake fat bombs are ideal when you are craving for something sweet. They cater to your taste buds, and you don't have to sacrifice flavor or taste. Moreover, they are creamy and fluffy.

Ingredients for cheese fat bomb in bacon

a) butter melted (or heavy cream)
b) 3 oz. coconut oil room temp (or heavy cream*)
c) 3 tablespoons erythritol
d) 2 tbsp. vanilla extract
e) Baking chocolate
f) Cream cheese

Instructions

Put the ingredients in a mixing bowl. Use an electric mixer to mix the ingredients thoroughly. Continue mixing for 2-3 minutes.

Scoop the mixer into a cupcake pan and put it in the fridge for 2 hours. Alternatively, put the cupcake pan in the freezer for 30-40 minutes

Transfer the cupcake tins from the pan to air-tight containers and refrigerate for up to 2 weeks.

Nutritional Information

Keto Cheesecake Fat Bombs

Amount Per Serving (1 Fat Bomb (0 carbs!))
Calories 107   **% Daily Value***
1. **Fat** 15g   17%
2. **Cholesterol** 20mg   7%
3. **Sodium** 64mg   3%
4. **Potassium** 13mg   0%
5. **Carbohydrates** 0g   0%
6. Sugar 0g   0%
7. **Protein** 0g   0%
8. **Vitamin A** 245IU   5%
9. **Calcium** 10mg   1%
10. **Iron** 0mg
11. **Saturated fat**   40%

You also make keto cheddar cheese and bacon balls. The ingredients for this include 5 oz. bacon, 5 oz. cream cheese, 1 tbsp. butter, ½ tbsp. pepper and 5 oz. cheddar cheese. You can also add ½ tbsp. chili flakes if you like. Start by frying the bacon in butter until it is golden brown. Put it aside to cool. Cut the bacon in small pieces and put in a bowl. Fry the bacon. Mix the grease left, frying the bacon with the rest of the ingredients. Put the bowl for 15 minutes before shaping them into balls. Crumble the bacon. Make small sized balls and roll in the bacon. Ready to eat.

Notes

Use any type of flavored cheese you like

If you do not like bacon, roll the cheese balls in chopped nuts, herbs, or cheese of your choice.

Alternatively, you can make fantastic low-carb bacon crab Rangoon. All you need to do is to get the right ingredients and proceed to soften the cream cheese. In a mixing bowl, mix the cream cheese with canned crab, seasoning, and shredded mozzarella. Mix until it becomes firm and put it in the fridge. Remove them from the fridge and roll in the bacon.

Bacon crab fat bombs are full of nutrients and flavor, which makes them suitable for all. In addition, they are keto and gluten-free. You are supposed to consume at least 70 percent of calories from fat while on a keto diet. Only 10 percent of your calories should come from carbohydrates and 15 percent proteins. You are not supposed to take fruit, vegetable, legumes, or grains. Many people have had success with the keto diet. It has helped many to lose weight because it is an easy regimen to follow. There are tons of options, and you will not feel hungry with all the great fat bomb options available. To make a bacon crab Rangoon fat bomb, you will need 1 packet of cream cheese,1 tbsp. of garlic powder, 1 can crab, pepper, slices of bacon, and salt, ☐ tbsp. garlic powder.

Instructions

- Start by softening the cream cheese. In a bowl, mix canned crab with minced garlic, mozzarella cheese, salt, pepper, and onion powder. Put in the fridge for 1 hour.
- Cook the bacon and chop into small pieces after it has cooled.
- Scoop 1 tbsp. of cream cheese and form them into ball shapes. Roll the ball in bacon and place it in the fridge for 30 minutes. Serve.

NEAPOLITAN FAT BOMBS

We can all remember the days we used to sit on the front door-step to hear the ice cream truck coming. Have you ever seen children racing to the track and how happy they are when they are given the frozen cups? It is magical, and that is exactly what happened. Neapolitan fat bombs are the best treats you can ever have. You can make them recreate childhood memories and eat on keto. While it is time consuming compared to other fat bomb treats, Neapolitan fat bombs are worth it. An added advantage with them is that there is plenty to choose from.

Ingredients

½ cup butter

½ cup cream cheese

½ cup of coconut oil

20 drops of stevia

½ sour cream

2tbps erythritol

1 tbsp. vanilla extract

2 strawberries

Instructions

- mix coconut oil, butter, sour cream, liquid stevia, erythritol, and cream cheese in a bowl.

-blend the ingredients using an immersion blender.

- put the mixtures in 3 different bowls, and in the second bowl, add cocoa powder.

-To the third bowl add vanilla extract. Mix the ingredients together properly and separate the chocolate mixture into a container. Pour the content into a fat bomb mold and put it in the fridge for 1 hour. When everything turns out as expected, you can do the same procedure with the vanilla extract and put it in the fridge. Proceed to freeze the vanilla mixture for 25 minutes and do the same with the vanilla mixture. Keep checking to see it is ready. Remove from the fat bomb molds when they are ready and serve.

You can never go wrong with keto fat bombs. You always go for keto Neapolitan fat bombs if you have nothing in mind. It is a simple recipe that anyone on a low-carb diet can adopt. You can opt for no-bake fat bombs with three layers including chocolate, fruit, and cream, which is savory and sweet. The traditional Neapolitan fat bomb consists of a layer of chocolate, vanilla, and strawberry. It is slightly sweet, but you can add strawberries to add more taste to it.

Many people prefer a mixture of berries in the Neapolitan ice cream. Anyone who desires to have a keto fat bomb needs to learn how it is made. If you are adding berries into the Neapolitan fat bombs, start by preparing the berry layer. Add all the ingredients in a pan and simmer for 5 minutes. Smash the mixture with a fork and pour the mixture into an ice cube mold. Mix erythritol, butter, and heavy cream in a pan to prepare the cream layer. Let it simmer until the mixture has completely melted. Use a fork to whisk the mixture until it is well combined. Once the mixture is ready, pour it on top of the berry layer and freeze for 30 minutes. Prep the chocolate layer by melting chocolate and coconut oil together. Pour in the first two layers of the mixture and let it freeze overnight. Serve.

Neapolitan fat bombs	fats	calories	carbs	fiber	Net carbs	protein
½ cup butter	92	814	0.07	0	0.07	0.13

½ cup sour cream	22.25	228	5	0	5	2.81
½ cup coconut oil	107.98	972	0	0	0	0
½ cream cheese	39.95	405	6	0	6	7
½ tbsp. erythritol	0	0	0	0	0	0
Medium strawberries	0.07	8	1.8	1.8	0.5	0.16
1 tbsp. vanilla	0	13	0.5	0	0.5	0
20 drops of liquid stevia	0	0	0	0	0	0
Total	263.80	2565	20.50	4.5	16.91	12.40

This treat can be taken with other meals. Fat bomb snacks go along with the Keto diet because they add a taste to plain dishes. Eating plain food is boring, and fat bombs allow you to switch things up.

When people hear about the fat bomb breakfast for keto, they have mixed feelings about it. Some think that it cannot be tasty while others are not interested in trying it out. The truth of the matter is that fat bombs for keto are the best option one could once. It not only full of nutrients but also easy to make. To make breakfast fat bombs in bacon, you will need ¼ avocado, 1 hard-boiled egg, ¼ lime juice. 1 tbsp. Mayonnaise, 5 cooked bacon slices, 4 tbsp. butter, and a dash of salt.

Instructions

- Mix together the hardboiled egg, butter, mayonnaise, avocado, cilantro, and pepper. Mash the ingredients using a fork to have a smooth paste. Season with pepper and salt and then add a juice of a lime.
- Fry the bacon and keep 2 tablespoons of bacon grease. Add the grease to the first mixture and stir. Put in the fridge for 1 hour. Separate the bacon into small pieces in a bowl.
- Form the fat bomb into small balls and add them to the

bacon. Serve.

Notes

If you don't have time, buy hardboiled eggs to save time spent in boiling them. Otherwise, if you have time, put eggs in a pot and add water to cover them. Let the eggs boil for 12 minutes and drain the water.

Put the boiled eggs into an ice bath and let it cool before peeling. Don't mind if you have a hard time peeling the eggs because they are slightly harder to peel than older eggs.

References

Abraham, L. (2019, April 25). Cookie Dough Keto Fat Bombs. Retrieved from https://www.delish.com/cooking/recipe-ideas/a19756323/cookie-dough-keto-fat-bombs-recipe/

CHAPTER 6: BUNS

In most parts of the world, almost every meal we have is somehow made from wheat. A bun is a tiny, can be sweet, an item made from bread. They can exist in different sizes and also shapes. In most cases, they are almost equal to the size of a hand. To make a ketogenic bun, we use most of the time a cloud bread. This works well in a making bun. We use cloud bread because it contains a very small amount of carbs. Let's look at how we can prepare this delicacy of keto burger buns for use in weight loss. This homemade low carb bun is gluten-free. This recipe gives us soft texture keto burger buns. This recipe does not use either eggs or any yeast. Instead, we use almond flour and coconut flour. These buns can be also be used in a paleo burger.

You can use the buns just after baking, or you can slice them and toast them for about two minutes in an oven. This will add a fantastic crispy texture to our buns. Keto burger buns make very delicious cheeseburgers that a very low in carbs. You can store the burger buns since they do not have any eggs that can cause them to get spoiled. They can be stored for up to five days at the normal room temperature. It is also convenient to wrap them in a clean kitchen towel in order to keep them moist and, most importantly, fresh for consumption. The buns tend to become softer as time goes by. If you prefer them when they are crispy, you can use the toaster to bring the crispy felling back to life again. This will depend on your choice because some people like them when they are soft.

Ingredients

    i)   Baking soda -This is used in a no yeast keto

bun. We use baking powder to raise our dough, so as it just looks similar to an ordinary bun.

ii)   Almond -You can use almond meal or almond flour; this will still give you the best results.

iii)   Coconut flour -Using coconut flour is a little bit tricky. It is tricky because you have to ensure your coconut flour is highly sifted. It is also highly advisable to measure the flour in grams instead of using a cup for better precision.

iv)   Apple cider vinegar -Since this recipe does not contain any gluten, the purpose of the vinegar is to chemically react with our baking soda for the dough to rise. You can also use lemon juice if you happen not to possess the apple cider vinegar.

v)   Ground psyllium husk -this is the magician in this simple recipe. Most bakers advise that you don't use any other alternative to this because it plays an essential role in our recipe.

vi)   Olive oil -If you do not have olive oil, you can use any vegetable oil of your own choice.

Procedure for preparing keto burger buns:

i)   Firstly, heat an oven to 200° C. This is the appropriate temperature for baking our buns.

ii)   Use a parchment paper to cover your baking tray that you are going to use. Spray some oil on the surface of the parchment paper. This will prevent the dough from sticking on your parchment paper.

iii)   Measure the required ingredients depending on how many buns you want to prepare. These ingredients should be placed in different and separate containers.

iv)   Place all of your dry ingredients in an enormous bowl and stir them until they combine entirely with each other.

v) Add the other ingredients to the dry mixture. Apple cider vinegar, water, olive oil, and baking powder should all be added at this particular step.

vi) Mix the ingredients vigorously using a kitchen spatula for a half a minute. After this, you can proceed to use your own hands to knead the ingredients into a dough for one minute. You should note that when you are beginning the kneading, the mixture will be somehow liquid. It will start to harden as you continue. The dough will be formed after approximately one and a half minutes into kneading. So, you have to be patient during this period.

vii) Take all the dough and form a sphere. This sphere will be very soft and moist. Put this dough in a bowl for some ten minutes. This will give the psyllium husks time to absorb any extra moisture and make an elastic tender dough, which is what we actually want.

viii) Knead the dough for another half a minute and separate it into six equal parts.

ix) Make each part into a ball.

x) Put the ball on the baking tray you have prepared earlier. The distance between each ball should be equal to the length of one human thumb. We give them this distance so that they do not touch each other while we are baking.

xi) Apply some pressure on top of the ball to give them a beautiful burger bun shape.

xii) Apply a small amount of water on each ball and add some little sesame seeds. The sesame seed will stick on the ball, and they tend to give it a crispy feeling at the same time they remain soft in the middle.

xiii) Bake the dough for about twenty to twenty-five minutes. The dough should be in the middle of the oven. When it is ready, the top of the dough will be brown and dark, without forgetting that it will also be crispy.

xiv)   Take the dough out of the oven and place it on a cooling rack for about twenty minutes.

xv)   Finally, our keto burger bun is ready, now slice it into two halves with a bread knife. You can toast the inside of the bun in any grill mode. You do this in order to make the center of the burn to be crispy. It is highly recommended to add cheddar cheese on the surface of each half. Bake again until all the cheese melts.

One of the common myths many people in the world have is that they believe the first hamburger was made in Hamburg. This is a place located in Germany. It is somehow true because the idea came from Hamburg, Germany. This is the reason why it is called Hamburg because of the birthplace of the concept. The hamburger sandwich was invented sometime later. It gained its popularity because of the beef they were made up of. This beef was from cows that were being raised in the countryside.

This beef was chopped and added some spices and formed into patties. During this time, there was no technology for refrigeration, so fresh meat has to be cooked instantly. Due to its popularity, the price of beef hamburgers rose by a considerable amount. This led to the beef being replaced by other expensive types of beef. After some of the Germans migrated into the United States of America, they brought together with them their culture. This culture also included their hamburger recipe. Some of them started cafes and restaurants in the major big cities such as Chicago.

It did not take a lot of time for the hamburger to be accepted by the Americans into their daily life menu. This is the point where the connection between the German hamburger and the U.S.

hamburger ends. The difference between the two is only one. This is the introduction of buns. These two pieces of bread became famous with time within the people at that time. People who were working nearby will order food. The food that they order is served to them through a window, and they ate the food very fast to get back to their work. This will later evolve into the present food carts. These food carts introduced the beef into their hamburgers. This was liked by most customers.

Since Hamburg has already proven to be difficult to eat while standing, this led to the introduction of the two slices of bread. It completely solved this problem, and hence the sandwich hamburger was born. A low carb hamburger is a very convenient way to reduce weight without changing our eating habits by a large percentage. This will only change the flavor of the burger to a new and better taste, and this is what we want in life, to experience new things without harming our health and wellbeing. We that in mind, we shall now look at how we can prepare this fast food. We are going to call it fast food because it takes very little time to make.

The recipe that we will be using is a keto recipe, meaning our hamburger will contain a very small amount of carbs. The recipe below contains very a very low count of carbs. This recipe takes about ten minutes for preparation and thirteen minutes for cooking. It takes a total of twenty-three minutes to prepare the keto hamburger buns fully.

Ingredients.

i)   2 Oz of cream cheese.

ii)   1 metal plate for baking a cake. You can also use a pan, but there is no need to worry a lot about where you can place the dough for baking.

iii)   2 tablespoons of oat fiber -You can also use the protein powder in place of oat or almond flour.

iv)   1 big and healthy egg.

v)   ¼ cup of some sifted quality almond flour.

vi)   1 tablespoon of baking powder –You can use baking powder and not yeast.

vii)   ½ cup cheese of skim grated mozzarella.

Below is the procedure that you are going to follow (the steps are well explained for easy understanding and implementation)

- Take the mozzarella cheese together with cream cheese and place them in a bowl. Heat the bowl in a microwave for some sixty seconds. While you are heating, try to stir the mixture in an interval of half a minute, this means that you are going to stir that mixture twice during the heating. After heating, remove the mozzarella cheese and cream cheese and with the egg into a food processing machine until they are smooth.
- Take all of your dry ingredients and add them to the mixture. Process the mixture until the mixture becomes a dough. This dough will be sticky, so there is no need to worry if this happens. If it happens to be too sticky to process, try leaving it for a couple of minutes, and continue processing.
- Heat the oven you are going to use to a temperature of about 400 F. Then put your rack right at the center of our oven. Use a parchment sheet to line your baking container. You can also use a metal pan, but you have to place it in the lowest part of the oven.
- Segment the dough into five pieces, which are of the same size each. Use oil on your hand and also the pieces, then mold each piece into a spherical ball. Place these balls on the parchment paper. Apply some little pressure on the balls using your hands but still making sure that they retain their shape.
- Take some ice cubes and put them on the pan at

- the bottom of our oven. You can use at least six ice cubes. After placing your balls in the oven, this will help the dough to rise and occupy more space.
- Bake your balls for about twelve minutes at 400 F. Continue baking until the balls are browned on the surface. The balls will be tender. Take them out and allow them to cool for some minutes. After cooling, you can now remove them from your baking sheet. Cooling the hamburgers gives them a temperature that allows for storage in a refrigerator.
- While in the refrigerator, they are supposed to be stored in an airtight container. They can be kept for seven to ten days without spoiling. You can also freeze them. In order to enjoy them, we have to heat them first.

A hot dog can be placed in a piece of bacon. Cheese can be added then sprinkled with some ketchup sauce and some specific type of chili. This has always been one of the staple foods in most of the American countries up to date. Many of the people are not curious enough to seek how it is made or what it contains. A hot dog is not an American idea.

It was conceived in a different part of the world according to its history. It was invented even before the great Christopher Columbus had started his journey to discover the most interesting part of the world. Before we dive into a hoe, this delicacy can be used to enhance weight loss, and let us first look at how its components came to an end up together. The hot dog sausage has its roots from the first century A.D. With time, and it has spread to different parts of the world. It first came to Europe in Germany. In this country, it was highly accepted by German culture. Up to the present day, some of the towns like Frankfurt claim to be the original creator.

The question remains how did it reach the U.S.? The German immigrants are responsible for the introduction of hotdog sausage into the U.S. Once it was introduced in the U.S., it was commonly referred to as "dachshund sausage." A German immigrant sold it on a food cart on the streets of New York City. This happens in the 1860s.

The main issue with hot dogs is that they have a lot of calories that contribute to weight gain. This is a scary situation for the enthusiasts who are in a diet of losing weight. There is no need to panic because there is already a recipe that is low in carbs and enhances the loss of weight. This recipe is mainly focused on how to bake keto hotdogs that are very low in carbs. Below is the list of ingredients and the procedure to combine the ingredients to obtain a low cab hotdog bun without a struggle or any kind of hustle. When these steps are carefully followed, and the instructions are adhered to, you will surely get an efficient keto hotdog bun. The amount of carbs in this recipe is one percent of the total carbs found in a standard hotdog bun.

Ingredients.

1. 3 fresh whites from a healthy egg.
2. 1 teaspoon of sea salt.
3. 1 ¼ cups of sifted almond flour.
4. 2 teaspoon of baking powder.
5. 1 ¼ cup of boiling water.
6. 2 teaspoon of cider vinegar. You can also use white wine vinegar in place of the cider vinegar.
7. 5 teaspoons of grounded psyllium husk powder.

Procedure

i) Heat up an oven to a temperature of 75° C. Place all of your moisture-free ingredients in a bowl and mix them properly.

ii) Heat water to boil. Add the egg whites and vinegar to the boiling water. To mix these ingredients, use the hand mixer for at least half a minute. Avoid altering the dough through over-mixing. This mixing should be consistent.

iii) Apply some water to your hands. Do this so that your hands are moist when handling the dough. Divide the dough into ten pieces. Roll these pieces into shapes of hotdog buns. While placing them on a baking sheet, make sure there is adequate space between each bun. You do this because when you bake, they tend to increase in size.

iv) Place your dough into the bottom rack of your oven. Bake for about forty to fifty minutes. There will be a hollow sound when you try to tap the lower part of the bun. Once this happens, it means your buns are ready.

v) Remove them from the oven and serve with high-quality hotdogs. The topping will depend on the person who is going to consume the keto hot-dog buns.

Almond buns are the best buns that can be baked using almond flour. Most of the people have tried using other flours in keto. The other flours are nothing compared to this kind of flour. These buns taste better and are also sugar-free. It means they automatically have a deficient percentage of carbs. When you compare the texture of these buns to the other buns, it is kind of dry than the others. This property makes it appropriate to be used in a toast. This recipe contains technical terms such as "pofiber."

This is basically fiber from dried potatoes. You can purchase from almost any online shop. After baking, these buns can be refrigerated. There are some recipes in which the end products cannot be refrigerated because the contents that are present can cause it to spoil. The recipe that we are going to be looking at is very simple, and you are not required to learn other recipes in order to perfect this one. The dough that is formed is very sticky. If you want to handle the dough efficiently, you will have to moist your hands first.

Ingredients.

- 2 teaspoons of sea salt.
- 60 grams of butter that is melted and cooled for a little time.
- 8 eggs
- 3 tablespoons of sesame seeds.
- 250 milligrams of almond flour.
- 300 milligrams of fat cottage cheese.
- 350 milliliters of pofiber.
- 2 teaspoons of baking powder.
- 3 tablespoons of psyllium husk fibers.

Procedure

1. Using a blender blend, both the eggs and the cottage cheese thoroughly. Add the melted butter too into the combination of eggs and cottage cheese.
2. Heat your oven. The temperature is supposed to be of about 180° C
3. Combine all the dry ingredients and whip properly.
4. Add the dry ingredients to the eggs. Knead until you obtain a sticky dough.
5. Divide the dough into the desired number of buns.
6. Place the buns on a baking pan lined with parchment that has been oiled. This oiling prevents the buns from sticking on to the baking pan.
7. Bake for at least fifteen minutes.
8. Allow the buns to cool before you serve or refrigerating.

References

Suazo, A. (n.d.-b). 45 Insanely Good Keto Fat Bomb Recipes [Blog post]. Retrieved from https://www.bulletproof.com/recipes/keto-recipes/fat-bombs-recipes-1b2b3c4b4t/

Livermore, S. (2019, May 25). 13 Keto Fat Bombs That Will Make Snacking Way Less Stressful [Blog post]. Retrieved from https://www.delish.com/cooking/g4845/keto-fat-bomb-recipes/

CHAPTER 7: COOKIES AND ROLLS

If you've been scared of having any flour products since consuming them would most likely make you add weight, worry no more! This chapter covers amazing Keto friendly cookies and rolls, delicious, easy to make. And, most importantly, healthy.

These recipes will favor both the Keto and Non-Keto eaters; Keto cookies and rolls aren't as boring as many people think! The good thing about these amazing recipes is that you get to prepare them in very little time, and you can even carry them to work or school and have a healthy bite instead of diving into junk. It is hard saying goodbye to muffins, but these Keto rolls and cookies will satisfy all your sugar needs.

CRISSCROSS COOKIES BAKED IN THE OVEN

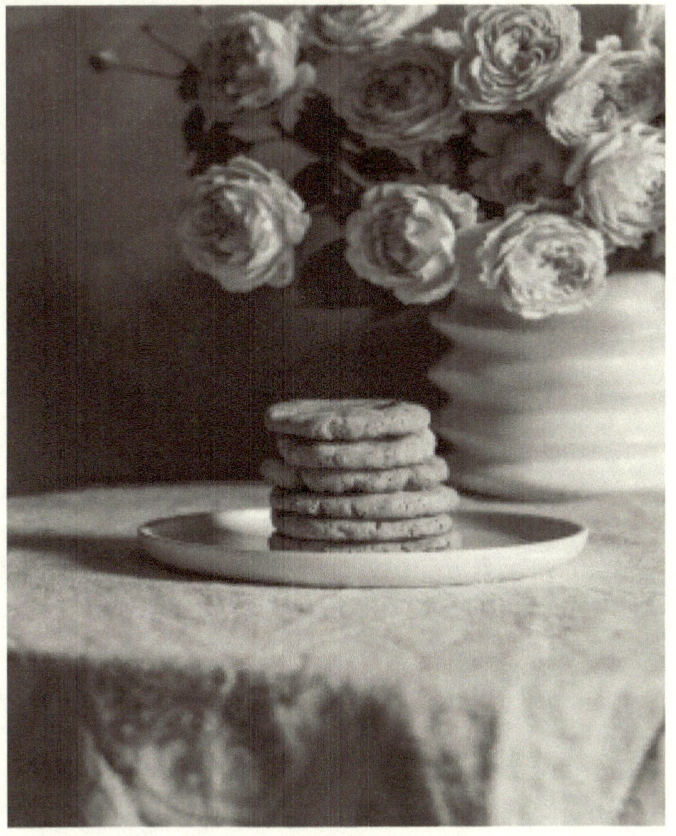

The crisscross cookies baked in the oven is one of the easiest cookie recipes ever! You use Four ingredients, and interestingly, you don't need eggs. These are very versatile cookies; they can be served with tea or at brunch or eaten as a dessert. You can also choose to use different dressings, i.e., almond or lemon extract, sprinkling them with cinnamon, or topping them up with blueberry jam to get healthy Keto cookies during the Christmas festivities.

Total Preparation & Cooking Time: 20 Minutes

Yields: 20 Servings

Nutritional Facts: Calories 100| Net Carb: 1g| Sugars: 0.5g| Fiber 1g| Protein 2g

Ingredients:

2 cups almond flour, blanched

½ cup erythritol, powdered or 6tbsp. Swerve sweetener

6 tbsp. butter, salted and softened

1 tsp vanilla extract

Instructions

1) The oven should be preheated to 350 F. Use a baking mat or parchment paper to line the baking sheet.
2) Combine the four ingredients in a bowl and stir thoroughly to form a cohesive dough. Ensure that the butter is soft enough to make it easier while stirring. Alternatively, you can use your hands to mix the ingredients.
3) Subdivide the dough to form 2o cookie balls. Place them on the lined baking sheet. They should be placed 2 inches from each other.
4) Use a fork to flatten the dough balls individually. Rotate the baking sheet at 90 degrees and flatten using the fork again; this step is what forms the crisscross pattern. Note that these cookies don't spread during baking; you mold them to the desired shape before baking.
5) Put the cookie balls in the oven for about 10 minutes, until they brown around the edges.
6) They should be soft when you take them out of the oven. Allow the cookies to cool. Transfer the cookies from the cookie sheet to the platter.

7) Serve and enjoy

Notes:
1) Storage of leftovers should be in airtight containers for a maximum of 5 days at room temperature.
2) The softened butter is very crucial in this recipe since it binds all the ingredients together. To avoid adding salt separately to your cookies, use salted butter.
3) There are many brands of sweeteners that you can use in your Keto recipe. Given that you are observing a Keto lifestyle, always make sure you a low carb sweetener. The Swerve sweetener is a good choice since it's also available in the version of the brown sugar, which goes perfectly with cookies. You may need to reduce the sweeteners depending on the percentage of sugar in the same.
4) You can do everything by hand; this includes forming the balls and mixing the ingredients. All you require is a wooden spoon and a mixing bowl. Equipment like the electric mixer isn't needed.
5) The determining factor of the baking time is the thickness and size of your cookies.
6) The crisscross cookies are ready if they have a texture that is short-bread like and crisp.

Some flavor mix-ins that can make your cookies more delicious:

- Substituting a portion of the vanilla extract with lemon or almond extract
- Substituting a portion of the flour with ground pecans, finely ground
- Adding shredded coconut or slice and toasted almonds
- Adding unsweetened cocoa powder or baking chocolate

- Adding fresh zest or juice from lemons

CHOCOLATE CHIP COOKIES

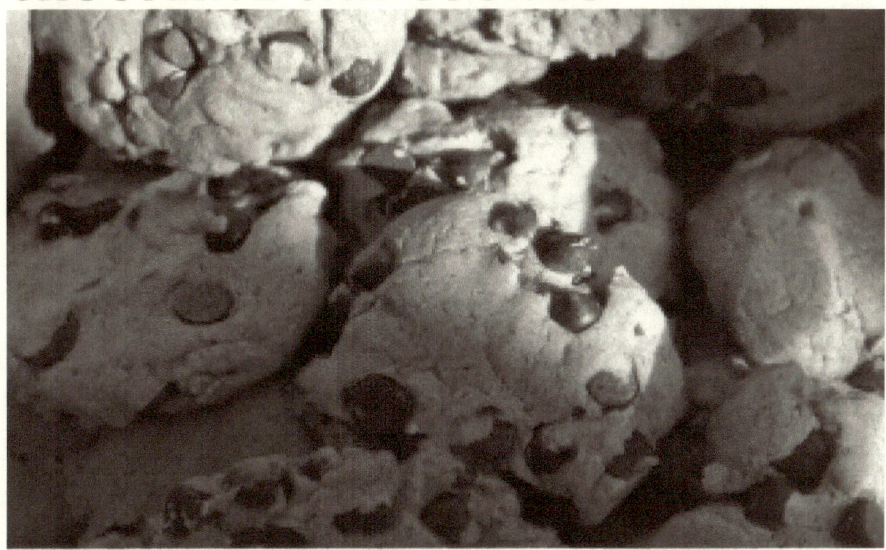

The Keto chocolate chip cookies recipe is easy to make, mixing all ingredients in one bowl and following very simple steps. These are kid-approved Keto cookies, which makes them a suitable and healthy snack for the whole family. You don't have to feel guilty every time you have a bite of your Keto chocolate chip cookie.

Total Cooking & Prep Time: 25 Minutes, Rest Time: 20 Minutes

Nutritional Facts: Calories: 180kcal

Yields: 6 Servings

Ingredients:

3 tbsps. butter, unsalted

½ tsp sweetener (stevia glycerite)

½ tsp vanilla extract

1 medium egg

¾ cup almond flour, blanched

1/8 tsp of salt (kosher)

Baking soda, 1/8 tsp

¼ cup of chocolate chips, dark

Instructions:

1)   Preheating of the oven should be at degrees F. Use parchment for lining the cookie/baking sheet.
2) Whip the egg, vanilla, Stevia, and butter together using an electric whisk. Make sure you incorporate these ingredients well.
3) Add the almond flour gradually until well mixed. Then add the salt and baking soda and mix.
4)   Use a spatula to fold the dark chocolate chips into the mixture.
5)   Place the mixed dough on the lined cookie sheet (scoop using rounded tablespoons, two inches apart). Use your hand to flatten the dough gently.
6)   Bake the Keto chocolate chip cookies for approximately 14 minutes, until golden brown. Be sure to check after twelve minutes to ensure that they don't burn.
7)   Allow the cookies to rest for approximately 20 minutes.
8) Serve and enjoy!

Notes:

1)   Use blanched almond flour, finely ground instead of almond meal to get wonderfully light chocolate chip cookies.

2)   You can use granulated sweeteners if you don't have stevia glycerite

3)   There are many brands of sweeteners that you can use in your Keto recipe. Given that you are observing a Keto lifestyle, always make sure you a low carb sweetener. The Swerve sweetener is a good choice since it's also available in the version of the brown sugar, which goes perfectly with cookies. You may need to reduce the sweeteners depending on the percentage of sugar in the same.

4)   Allow your cookies to cool on the cookie sheet, not on the cooling rack; this ensures that they become crunchy upon cooling

5)   You can store the Keto chocolate cookies safely in airtight containers for a maximum of 5 days.

PEANUT BUTTER COOKIES

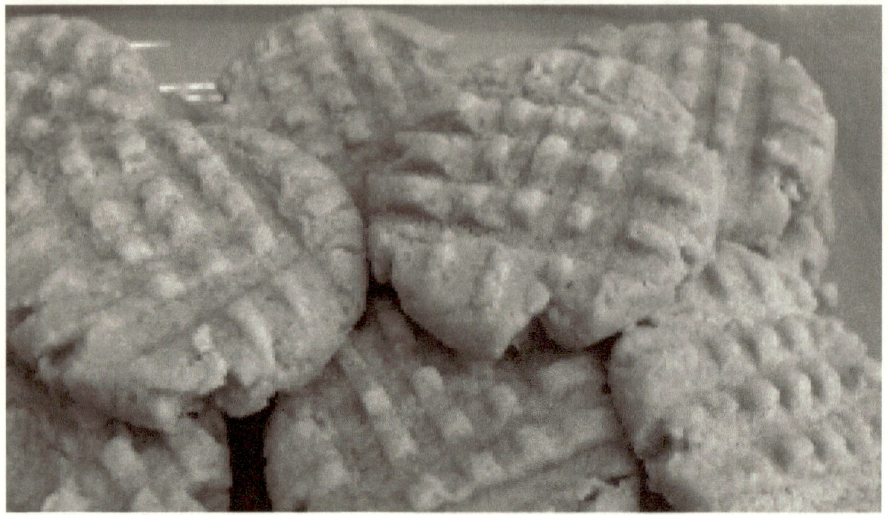

Total Preparation & Cooking Time: 1 Hour

Yields: 10 Servings

Nutrition Facts Per Serving: Calories: 195| Fat 16.9g26%| Carbs 5.7g2%| Protein 6.5g13%| Fiber 2.6g10%

Ingredients

Filling (Peanut Butter)

¼ cup peanut butter, creamy

¾ tbsp. butter

1 ½ tbsp. Swerve Sweetener, powdered

Chocolate Cookies

Almond flour, ¾ cup

Cocoa powder, 3 tbsps.

Grass-fed gelatin, 1 tbsp.

½ tsp of baking powder

½ tsp of salt

1 egg

¼ cup softened butter

¼ cup almond butter, creamy

½ cup of Swerve Sweetener

½ tsp of vanilla extract

Instructions:

Filling (Peanut Butter)

1) Use parchment or waxed paper to line the cookie sheet.
2) Place the butter and peanut butter in a bowl that is microwave safe. Melt them on high temperature, stirring until it becomes smooth. Upon melting, add the sweetener and whisk until all lumps dissolve.
3) Use about a tablespoon at a time to drop the mixture on the lined cookie sheet to create little patties. Place the baking sheet in a freezer for approximately 1 hour.

Note: If the mixture is excessively runny, add 1-2 tablespoons of Swerve sweetener to thicken it.

Chocolate Cookies

1) Preheating of the oven should be at 350 degrees F. Use parchment papers or silicone mats for lining the baking sheets.
2) Whisk the baking soda, salt, gelatin, cocoa powder, and almond flour in a large bowl.
3) In a different bowl, beat the Swerve sweetener, butter,

and almond butter together, ensuring that they mix properly. Beat in the egg and add the vanilla extract. Add the flour, beating it into the mixture until everything comes together.

4)   Scoop one tablespoon of dough into a patty, one at a time. Place one of the frozen patties on top, cover with another tbsp. of dough. Seal the edges. Repeat this procedure until you exhaust the remaining frozen patties and dough.

5)   Place the cookies with the peanut filling on the lined baking sheets, leaving a space of approximately 2 inches between them

6)   Bake for approximately 12-16 minutes, until they puff up.

7)   Allow to cool on the pan and serve.

Notes:

1)   You should prepare the frozen patties before making the dough.

2)   The peanut butter mixture shouldn't be super runny but drippy. Adding more sweetener will help in thickening a mixture that is too runny.

3)   There are many brands of sweeteners that you can use in your Keto recipe. Given that you are observing a Keto lifestyle, always make sure you a low carb sweetener. The Swerve sweetener is a good choice since it's also available in the version of the brown sugar, which goes perfectly with cookies. You may need to reduce the sweeteners depending on the percentage of sugar in the same.

4)   Storing of Keto peanut butter cookies should be at room temperature; this helps to retain the chewy consistency. Always store them in airtight containers. Alternatively, you can store them in a refrigerator; allow them to get to room temperatures before serving.

SNICKERDOODLES COOKIES

This easy recipe with straight forward steps will yield lightly tangy and perfectly soft Keto and gluten-free cookies. These snickerdoodles cookies are slightly chewy and crispy, which gives them such an exciting combination of textures and tastes. The coating of the sweetener and cinnamon makes these snickerdoodles cookies perfect, especially if taken with a cup of hot coffee!

Total Preparation & Cooking Time: 30 Minutes

Yields: 12 Servings

Nutritional Facts: 68KCAL

Ingredients:

60 g of almond flour

1/4 tsp cream of tartar

8 g coconut flour

¼ tsp baking soda

¼ tsp salt, kosher

1 egg

56 g unsalted butter (grass-fed), at room temperature

1/4 cup of allulose or erythritol xylitol to taste

¾ tsp vanilla extract

¼ tsp xanthan gum

Cinnamon Sugar

1 tsp cinnamon

1 tbsp. allulose or xylitol

Instructions:

1) The preheating of the oven should be at 190°C/375°F. Use baking mats or parchment papers to line the baking trays
2) Add cream of tartar, baking soda, salt, almond flour, xanthan gum, and coconut flour to a bowl. Whisk thoroughly. Set aside.
3) In a separate bowl, use an electric mixer to cream butter until it softens. Add the sweetener as you continue to mix until fluffy and light (approximately 8 minutes).
4) Add the egg and vanilla extract, mixing until it begins to be incorporated; the consistency should be slightly broken. Set your mixer on low, pour in half the flour mixture, mixing gradually. Pour the remaining half and mix.
5) Use a tablespoon to scoop out small cookie rounds. Roll in the mixture of cinnamon sugar and flatten slightly.
6) Transfer the scooped cookies to the lined tray. Place in the oven and bake for approximately 7-8 minutes, until they turn to a golden brown color.
7) Allow the cookies to cool for 15 minutes
8) Serve and enjoy

Notes:

1) If you prefer your Keto snickerdoodles softer and thicker, avoid flattening them excessively as this will determine their end texture.
2) There are many brands of sweeteners that you can use in your Keto recipe. Given that you are observing a

Keto lifestyle, always make sure you a low carb sweetener. The Swerve sweetener is a good choice since it's also available in the version of the brown sugar, which goes perfectly with cookies. You may need to reduce the sweeteners depending on the percentage of sugar in the same.

3)   Storage of the snickerdoodles cookies shouldn't exceed five days in airtight containers. You can freeze the pre-shaped dough for three months. Thaw them outside the fried overnight and pass them through cinnamon sugar before baking, when you need them.

4)   You can also freeze these cookies for preservation. Allow them to thaw before consumption.

CHOCOLATE FAT KETO COOKIES

The chocolate fat Keto cookies are perfect dessert items in menus for people observing the Keto diet, low in carbs! They have a tantalizing taste, especially when completed with the sugar-free chocolate dipping. They come loaded with chocolate chip cookies, which makes it a favorite for cookie lovers, observing healthy eating habits. They are delicious and easy to make and are the perfect pick for your afternoon snack.

Total Preparation & Chilling Time: 45 Minutes

Yields: 15 portions

Nutritional Facts: 137kcal|Fat:11g| Cholesterol:8mg| Saturated Fat: 5g| Protein:2g|Vitamin A: 95IU| Fiber:1g

Ingredients:

¼ cup softened butter

½ cup Erythritol sweetener (Swerve Sweetener)

¼ tsp vanilla extract, pure

1 cup almond flour

½ tsp salt, kosher

5 ounces Lily's dark chocolate chips

4 Ounces Hershey's chocolate chips (sugar-free)

Instructions

1) Beat butter until fluffy and light using an electric hand mixer until fluffy and light. Add vanilla, salt, and sugar. Mix well.

2)   Add flour, little by a little while mixing until you achieve the dough consistency.

3)   Add the dark chocolate chips, mix and use a plastic wrap to cover. Refrigerate for approximately 15 minutes.

4) Remove the dough from the fridge. Scoop 1-inch balls of the dough using a tablespoon or cookie scoop. Place the balls on a lined baking sheet (use parchment paper to line the rimmed baking sheet)

5)   Put the chocolate chips (sugar-free) in a microwave-friendly dish. Put in the microwave and keep stirring in 30 seconds intervals until smooth.

6)   Dip the chilled fat balls in the melted chocolate. Return them to the baking sheet. Freeze them for approximately 5 minutes, until the chocolate hardens.

7) Serve and enjoy

Notes:

1)   The carbs listing for each fat cookie is 12 grams.

2)   The Swerve Sweetener and dark chocolate chips contain Erythritol, while the sugar-free chocolate chips contain Maltitol.

3)   There are many brands of sweeteners that you can use in your Keto recipe. Given that you are observing a Keto lifestyle, always make sure you a low carb sweetener. The Swerve sweetener is a good choice since it's also available in the version of the brown sugar, which goes perfectly with cookies. You may need to reduce the sweeteners depending on the percentage of sugar in the same.

4)   Storing of chocolate fat Keto cookies should be done in airtight containers, refrigerated for a maximum of 2 weeks.

KETO LOW CARB ROLLS

These Keto low carb rolls recipe yield soft rolls that are sugar and gluten-free, and low in carbs. They are made using yeast, which makes them extra fluffy and pillow-light. They are an excellent choice for breakfast, and they also go well as low carb rolls with dinner or lunch.

Total Preparation and Cooking Time: 35 Minutes

Yields: 16 Servings

Nutritional Facts: Calories 257

Ingredients

    1)   Dry Ingredients

400 g or 4 cups of ground almonds or almond flour

2 tbsp. baking powder

6 tbsp. protein powder(whey)

2tbsp. inulin

4 tsp dry yeast(active)

6 tbsp. husk powder(psyllium)

    2)   Wet Ingredients

4 large eggs, at room temperature

100 g /1/2 cup of melted butter

Egg whites (4) at room temperature

60 ml of lukewarm water

100g yogurt, Greek

Instructions:

1)   Put the inulin and yeast into a bowl. Add the luke-warm water; it should be warm when you touch it. Use a kitchen towel to cover the bowl. Leave it for approximately 10 minutes in a warm place until it begins to thicken and froth.

2)   Combine the baking powder, husk powder, protein powder, and almond flour in a separate bowl. Set the bowl aside.

3)   Using a food processor or an electric mixer, whisk the egg whites and eggs (at room temperature), yeast mixture(yeast), and warm melted butter until they combine thoroughly.

4)   Add half of the mixture of the dry ingredients and yogurt. Process them until they mix well, add the remaining half of the mixture. The dough will become thick quickly since the almond flour, and the psyllium absorbs the moisture.

5)   Use parchment paper to line a casserole dish and pie dish. Wet your hands lightly and make sixteen dough balls. Leave some space between the balls as they will increase in size significantly.

6)   Use a kitchen towel and or a lightly oiled cling film to cover the casserole dish. Find a warm place and place the dish for about 1 hour until the rolls expand substantially (You could place the dish on top of the radiator)

7)   The oven should be preheated to 350 F towards the end of the one hour.

8)   Bake for approximately fifteen minutes until the rolls begin to brown. Cover with aluminum foil loosely and bake for an additional 10 minutes.

9)   Serve and enjoy.

Notes:

1) Don't be tempted to take shortcuts with the temperatures when dealing with the ingredients; yeast dies if the environment is too cold or too hot. Ensure that the water is warm, the melted butter is warm, and the eggs are at room temperature.

2) Ensure that you activate the yeast by proofing it; this is a very important step in this recipe. It must froth, bubble, and thicken. If it fails to do so, start the process of yeast activation afresh.

3) If you are in high altitude surroundings, preheat the oven to 375 F.

4) Storage of the low carb Keto rolls should be in moisture free and airtight containers, at room temperatures.

MOZZARELLA ROLLS

The Keto Mozzarella rolls recipe yields the perfect sandwich & dinner rolls in under 18 minutes. What's better than tasting the combined taste of the cream and mozzarella cheese in one roll? It's a recipe that is easy to do, and it's possible to store rolls can for five days, and they still retain their freshness.

Total Preparation & Cooking Time: 18 Minutes

Yields: 16

Nutritional Facts: Calories: 165| Fat: 13g| Carbs: 3g| Protein:10g| Sodium 104mg| Fiber 1g

Ingredients:

3 cups shredded mozzarella cheese

4 ounces cubed cream cheese

2 ½ cups almond flour

2 large eggs

4 tbsp. oat fiber or coconut flour

2 tsp baking soda

Instructions:

1) Put the cream and mozzarella cheese in a microwave-friendly bowl. Melt the cheese in the microwave for 1 minute at full power. Stir, heat the cheese for another 45 seconds. Scrape the mixture into a food processor and blend until it's mixed thoroughly. Add the eggs and blend.
2) Add all dried ingredients to the food processor bowl.

Process for approximately 10-15 minutes until thoroughly mixed.

3)   Cut a piece of cling film, spray it with oil. Scrape the dough onto the cling film. Since it's very sticky, shape it gently into a rectangular or disk shape. Place the wrapped dough in the freezer; this allows it to cool before putting it into the oven. (If the dough isn't excessively sticky, it doesn't need to be put into the freezer)

4)   The oven should be preheated to 400 degrees F. Place the rack in the middle part of the oven. Use a piece of a Silpat or parchment to line the cookie sheet.

5)   Take out the dough from the freezer when the oven is ready. Cut the dough into 16 pieces.

6)   Oil your hands lightly. Roll one portion of the dough gently to form a ball. Drop it on the lined cookie sheet; this flattens its' bottom. Repeat this process for the remaining pieces. You can sprinkle with dehydrated onion, poppy seeds, or sesame seeds, pressing into the dough gently; this allows the dough to adhere.

7)   Bake for about 12-14 minutes until the dough begins to brown and in some instances, split.

8)   Serve your Mozzarella rolls and enjoy!

Notes:

1)   Baking powder isn't a requirement in this recipe; the cream cheese contains an acid that reacts with baking soda making the rolls to rise. However, if your rolls fail to rise nicely, add 1 tablespoon of baking powder should be added.

2)   The texture of the Mozzarella rolls is a bit different from the typical rolls; it tends to be firm and a bit dry. Warming them before consumption helps in softening them up.

3)   Always check that you have preheated the oven to the

recommended temperature to ensure that your rolls rise as expected.

4)   Store the Mozzarella rolls in airtight, moisture-free containers. Room temperatures will enhance their longevity.

CINNAMON ROLLS

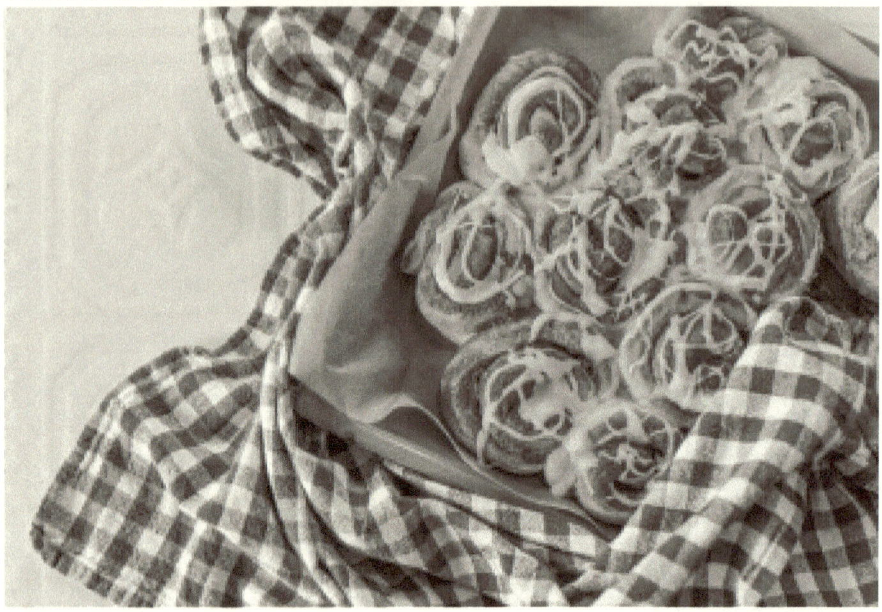

This Keto cinnamon rolls recipe fits the Low Carb style of living perfectly, and it comprises of the cream cheese frosting. It's simply irresistible. The amazing thing in the preparation of Keto Cinnamon rolls is that you don't have to wait for the dough to rise since yeast isn't a necessity! You can get this dough ready in less than 10 minutes, and the rolls are delicious!

Total Preparation and Cooking Time:

Yields: 30 Servings

Nutrition Facts: Calories: 85| Fat: 6.8g| Sodium: 217.5g|Cholesterol: 30.2mg|Total Carbs: 1.3g

Ingredients

4 cups of Mozzarella Cheese

1 ½ cups of almond flour

6tbsp. cream cheese

2tsp baking powder

2 eggs

2tsp cinnamon

2tbsp. Swerve or Stevia sweetener

¼ butter stick, melted

Ingredients for the Cheese Frosting

Heavy cream, 4 tsp

Cream cheese, 4 tsp

2tbsp. Swerve sweetener, powdered

Optional: ½ tsp of vanilla can be added to give it more flavor.

Instructions:

1) The cream cheese and Mozzarella cheese in a microwave-friendly bowl. Set the microwave on a high for approximately 1 minute. You can melt the cheese over a stove if you don't have a microwave on low heat.

2) After melting the cheese, add the eggs, baking powder, and almond flour. Save the stevia and cinnamon to sprinkle on the dough after rolling it out.

3) Stir the ingredients carefully until the mixture is smooth and well combined; this helps in cooling the dough a little.

4) At this point, the dough is very sticky. Place the dough on a parchment paper. Knead the dough continuously until all ingredients are completely mixed in. Sprinkling some coconut or almond flour on the dough when rolling it out prevents it from excessive sticking.

5)   Smoothen out the dough using a rolling pin into a big rectangle shape. Rolling the dough between 2 sheets of silicone parchment papers makes the rolling process easier.

6)   Melt the butter. Spread it over the rolled out dough, sparingly.

7)   Sprinkle Stevia sweetener and cinnamon over the dough

8)   Roll up the dough

9)   Use a string to divide the dough into 30 cinnamon rolls

10) Line the pan with a parchment paper before baking

11) Place the cinnamon rolls in the lined baking pan

12) Bake them for approximately 20 minutes in a 350 degrees oven until golden brown. The amount of baking time is dependent on the size of the rolls.

13) Begin mixing the frosting while the rolls are baking

14) Combine the powdered sweetener, cream cheese, and heavy cream into a large bowl. Set your mixer on high speed, mix the ingredients until smooth and nice.

15) Allow the rolls to cool. Apply the frosting.

16) Serve and enjoy.

Notes:

1)   Optional: You can sprinkle some pecans on top of the Keto cinnamon rolls.

2)   Storage of Keto cinnamon rolls should be in airtight, moisture-free containers at room temperature. They are safe for consumption for a maximum of 5 days.

3)   Be sure that the sweetener that you purchase adheres to the Keto diet requirements

4)   Never apply the frosting before the rolls cool

5)   Ensure that you have preheated your oven to the correct temperatures to ensure that your rolls rise properly.

References

Goodrum, T. (2018, August 16). 9 Keto Cookie Recipes That Are Somehow Part of a Diet [Blog post]. Retrieved from https://greatist.com/eat/keto-cookie-recipes#1

Lovefoodies. (2019). Crisscross Cookies. Retrieved from https://lovefoodies.com/crisscross-cookies/

CHAPTER 8: MUFFINS AND DONUTS

PEANUT BUTTER COOKIE MUFFINS

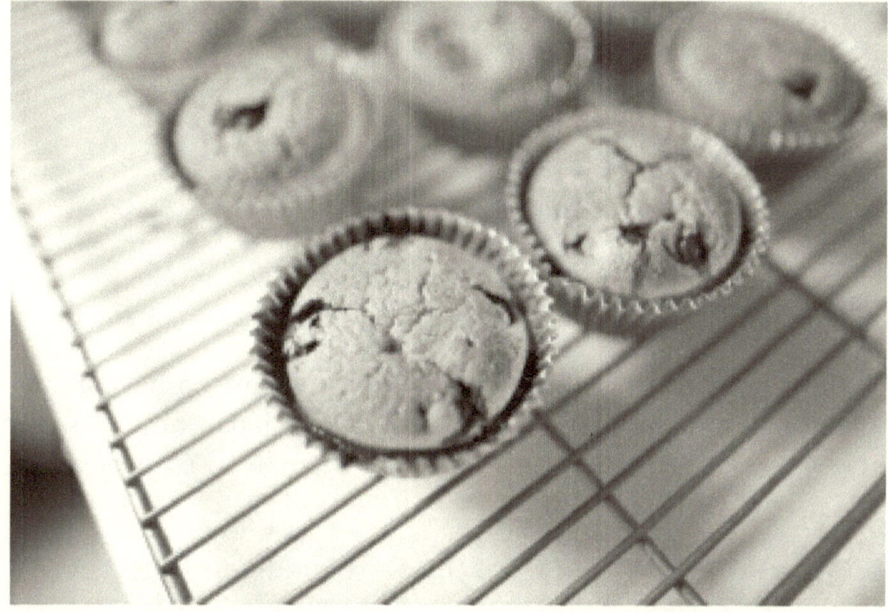

The preparation time is 20 min. The cooking time is 10-20 min, and a total time of 30 min

Ingredients

- Cooking spray-Coconut Oil
- Baking Blend THM 1 ½ cups
- Peanut flour pressed ¾ Cup
- Gentle Sweet ½ cup
- Baking powder 1 tbsp. – aluminum-free.
- ½ tsp. Salt
- Egg Whites 1 ½ cups
- Water 1 ½ cups
- Vanilla extract 1 ½ tsp.

- Chocolate Syrup-handy

Ingredients for Chocolate Syrup

- Water ½ cup

- Cocoa powder ¼ cup (unsweetened)

- Gentle Sweet 5 tbsp.

- Salt 3 pinches

- Vanilla extracts ½ tsp.

Instructions

1. Have your oven at 400 degrees. Next, ensure to have about 12 cups all with well put cupcake liners (well, parchment liners could work perfectly) and have your liners well sprayed with oil (coconut).

2. Ensure to then whisk all of the dry ingredients together in a sizable bowl. Next, have the wet or moist ingredients in and stir well and properly. Since the mixture will be quite wet, allow it for 10 minutes to first set up.

3. With that set and done, next ladle your batter onto every muffin cup and have them bake for 22 minutes. (In the meantime you could as well be preparing your chocolate syrup).

4. After your muffins have been well baked, have them removed from the baking tray/pan and allow them to cool for some time. Transfer then into a different tray and then gently drizzle the muffins with your then prepared chocolate syrup (if you have surplus syrup store in in the fridge maybe for future use on either pancakes or the same cupcakes).

Instructions for Syrup

Gather all your syrup ingredients and have them in the right proportions, then have them mixed in a saucepan and boil then over some heat (medium-high) as you occasionally whisk the mixture. After some time, lower your heat levels as you continue whisking gently and as your mixture simmers for several minutes. Now remove from heat/turn off the heat source.

Nutrition Facts

7g fats, 119 calories, 6mg cholesterol, 13g carbs (1g fiber & 3g sugars), 89mg sodium, 2g protein.

CREAMY PUMPKIN MUFFINS

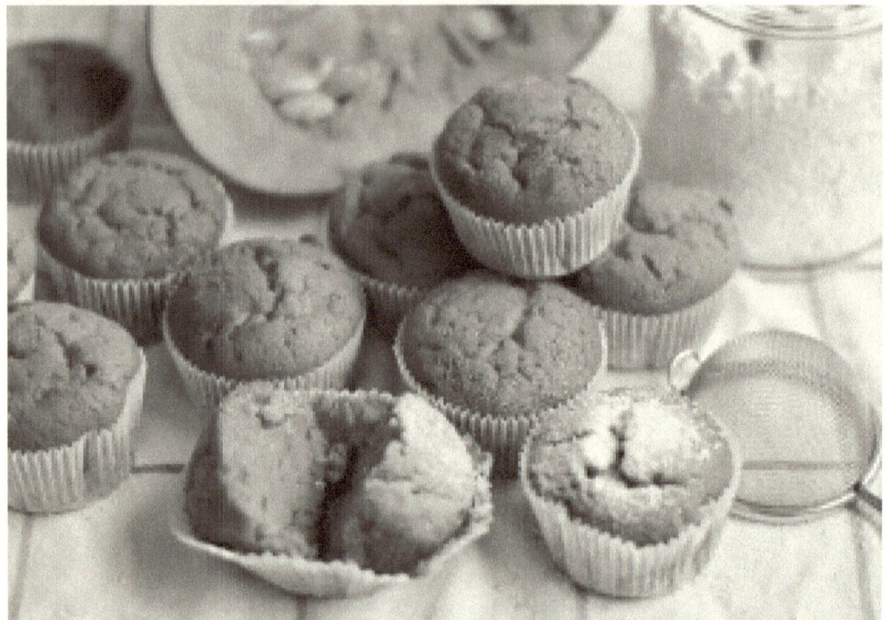

Produce: 12 pieces

Prepping Time: 10 min, Cooking Time: 20 min = Total Time: 30 min

Ingredients

- Softened butter half a cup
- Erythritol sweetener granulated one tablespoon & 2/3 cup, like Swerve
- Eggs (4 large)
- Pumpkin puree ¾ cup
- Vanilla extract 1 tsp.
- Almond flour one and a half cup

- Coconut flour half a cup

- Baking powder four teaspoons

- Pumpkin spice 2 tsp.

- Salt ½ teaspoon

- 8 oz. softened cream cheese

Instructions

1. Have your oven heated to about 350 degrees. Get a muffin pan or muffin cups and grease them or, better yet, have them lined.

2. Get a mixing bowl of your preference (depending on the number of pieces you want) cream your butter together with the sweetener (2/3 cup) until it is fluffy and light.

3. Put your eggs one after the other and combine them properly by a gentle mix.

4. Next, add in the vanilla and pumpkin puree and mix properly for an even combine.

5. Get yourself another bowl and put in the baking powder, salt, pumpkin spice, coconut flour, and almond flour and stir all together. Ensure to break any lumps that might form from either of the flours.

6. Having both mixtures separate, add your dry ingredients into the wet one and properly stir for an even combination. After a good mix, put the mixture into the already prepared muffin tray/tins.

7. Get another small bowl and stir in the sweetener (1tbsp) and the cream cheese (already softened). Put a well-filled tbsp. of the cream cheese on to

every muffin. To swirl your cream and the batter together, you could use a toothpick or a butter knife tip.

8. Have your art baking for about twenty to twenty-five minutes or better yet till a toothpick is completely spotless after being inserted into the center of the loaf. (Most preferable spot would be where it is less of the cheese cream and just muffin, this prevents you from confusing melted cream for undone batter).

Useful notes

- By any chance, if you get difficulties swirling in your cream mixture, have it heated/warmed in your microwave for approximately 10-20 seconds before you have it mixed.

- If you like them a bit chilled or at room temperature, it's allowed as well you can have them in a fridge in an airtight container.

Nutrition

2g proteins, 6g fiber, 4g sugar, 623mg carbs, 2g cholesterol, 11g trans-fat, 0g unsaturated fats, 99mg sodium

ZUCCHINI MUFFINS WITH CHOCOLATE CHIPS

Produce: 12 muffins

Prepping time of 15 min, Cooking time: 20 min = Total Time of 35 min

The Ingredients

- Unpeeled Zucchini & shredded two cups - (one small/medium)

- Ripe banana mashed ½ cup — about 4 ounces

- Coconut oil ¼ cup (melted & cool, light olive or canola oil)

- Honey ¼ cup

- brown sugar a quarter cup

- vanilla extract one tsp. - pure

- Eggs 2 large

- Cinnamon 1 tsp. and grounded

- Baking soda a half teaspoon

- A half teaspoon baking powder

- Salt ½ tsp.

- Wheat flour-whole & white two cups

- Chocolate chips 1/3 cups semi-sweet

Instructions

1. Get your oven to 375 degrees. Have your muffin tin greased lightly or lined using standard paper liners.

2. Having grated your zucchini, using a paper towel thoroughly squeeze to get rid of any excess water. If persistent, continue squeezing. If not already, get your coconut oil melted and allow it to cool to room temperature

3. Inside you, large bowl, get in your coconut oil, brown sugar, banana, and honey beat together until soft/smooth. Right after put in your eggs (previously at room temperatures) and properly mix until the mixture is well combined. (if the eggs are not at room temperature your oil- coconut may solidify).

4. Get the bicarbonate of soda, cinnamon, baking powder all with the salt on the batter then combine properly by mixing. Add in the flour by sprinkling then on low speed gently mix until id vanishes/disappears. Now using your hands (observe hygiene) fold in your zucchini together with the chocolate chips.

5. With the batter ready, scoop it into your muffin cups/tray (well prepared) and have them filled the only ¾ of the tin. Straight to your oven, bake them for the next 20-25 minutes. To know they are ready to insert your toothpick in which if it emerges spotless, it means your delicious work of art is ready. Have them removed from the baking unit and placed onto the wire rack. Allow it to cool down for about 5 minutes, then slowly lift your muffins out from the pan, and this time have them on the wire rack for complete cooling. (it prevents them from becoming soggy).

Helpful Recipe Note

- Have your muffins stored at room temperature, or as well, you can personally wrap them and have them frozen for some time till 3 months. You can let them thaw in the fridge overnight or unwrap then warm on little heat.

Nutrition Information

5g protein, 3g fiber, 14g sugar, 225mg potassium, 31g carbs, 8g fat, 5g saturated fat, 201 calories.

BRIEF MUFFINS

Prepping time of 10 min, the cooking time of 25 min = Total time: 35 min

12 servings

Essentials needed

- Flour all-purpose 2 cups
- 1 egg
- Baking powder 3 tsp.
- Salt ½ tsp.
- White sugar ¾ cup
- Milk one cup
- Oil-vegetable ¼ cup

Instructions

1. Have your oven heating at 400 degrees.

2. Get a big container/bowl and put in sugar, salt, flour, baking powder, and all together stir correctly. Create a well like a feature at the center. Using a smaller bowl, get your eggs beat using your fork then as well stir your milk in and the salad oil. Right inside your well put the small bowl's mixture inside, then mix it hastily and lightly as well using a fork till moistened. Dare not to beat. It makes your batter lumpy, afterward into muffin cups/trays that have been appropriately paper-lined.

3. Variations:
    a. Blueberry Muffin: Put in fresh blueberries (1cup).

    b. Raisin Muffin: Add raisins (finely chopped) 1 cup.

    c. Date Muffin: Add dates (finely chopped) 1 cup.

    d. Cheese Muffin: Add Sharp yellow cheese, grated 1 cup.

    e. Bacon Muffins: Cooked bacon, crisp ¼ cup folded, and broken to bits.

4. Have them baked in 25 minutes' time till golden.

Nutritional Facts

Sodium 233mg, cholesterol 17mg, calories 181, carbs 29.7g, fats 5.6g

CHOCOLATE CINNAMON DONUTS

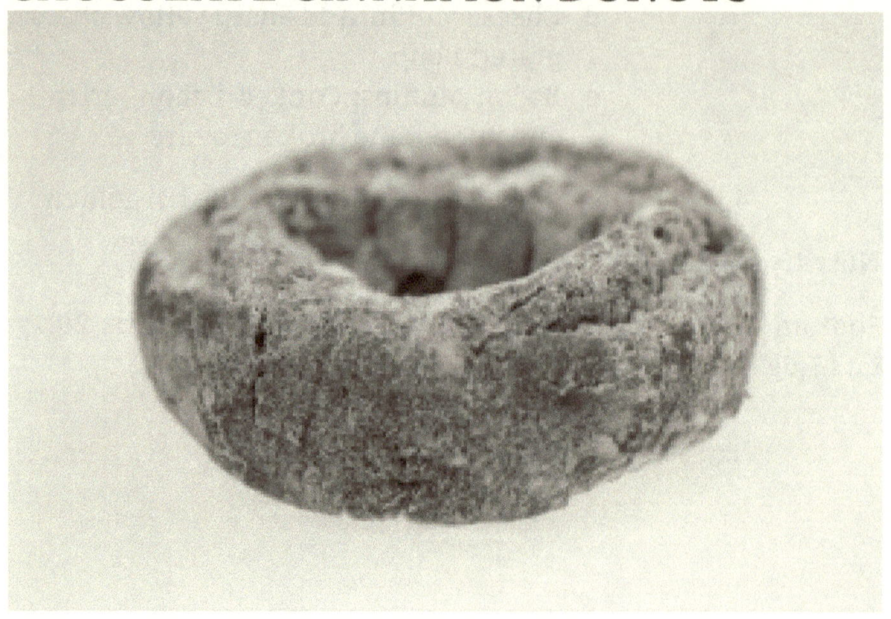

Prepping Time of 10 min Cooking time: 20 min = total time: 30 min

Essentials

- Coconut flour half a cup

- Erythritol ¼ cup or sweetener (low carb)

- Cocoa powder ¼ cup

- Eggs 6 & medium

- Coconut oil ¼ cup

- Coconut milk ¼ cup

- Cinnamon one tsp.

- Salt a quarter tsp.

- Baking soda ¼ tsp.

- Vanillas extract one tbsp.

Glaze:

- Unsalted butter 2 tbsp.

- Cinnamon 1 tbsp.

Instructions

1. Have your oven heated at 180C degrees.
2. In a bowl, put in your cocoa flour, salt, baking soda, cinnamon, and the erythritol and adequately mix.
3. Put in your coconut oil, vanilla extract, the eggs, and the coconut milk and thoroughly blend the mixture, ensuring you have no lumps insight or feel.
4. Get your donut molds and fill them with your prepared batter and have them baked for about 20 minutes till they are firm. Afterward, remove them and allow them to cool down.
5. Get your butter melted and add in your cinnamon then correctly mix.
6. Next thing, you directly immerse your donuts inside your cinnamon mixture.
7. Do you know what's next? Serve, smile, eat more, and enjoy!

Nutritional content:

Carbs 5g, calories 263, protein 8g, total carbs 12g, fiber 7g, fats 22g.

GLUTEN-FREE DONUT

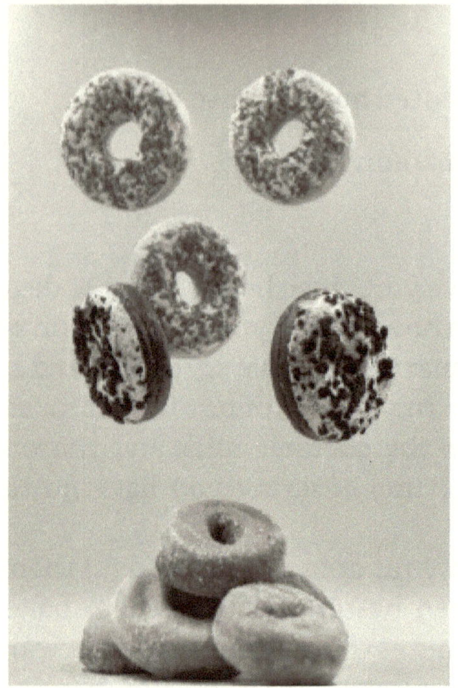

Recipe

It is all beautiful in baking some gluten-free donuts yourself!
— all, in addition, to satisfy your demanding donut craving all
and any moment you get one — imagine it better when you can
make a lot of them all with the right curves and rounds as you
like.

Prepping Time: 15 min & 30 min rise time, Cook Time: 1 min =
total time: one hour

Produce: 12 pieces

Ingredients:

- Flour-gluten free 3 2/3 cups

- Sugar-granulated ½ cup

- Bicarbonate of soda half a tsp.

- Salt one tsp.

- Cardamom-ground 1 tsp.

- Shortening ¼ mug

- Egg (1) & one egg yolk

- Milk 1 cup

- Vanilla paste 1 ½ tbsp. Or vanilla extract 5 tsp.

- Sugar-granulated 1 tbsp.

- Yeast (rapid rise) 2 ½ tbsp.

- Vegetable oil-high heat, for frying

- Confectioner's sugar all for dusting

Glaze:

- Confectioner's sugar one and a half cup
- Milk two to three tbsp.
- Vanilla extract teaspoon (one).

Chocolate glaze:

- Milk one tbsp.

- Cocoa powder 2 tbsp.

- Chocolate syrup 1 tbsp. (optional)

- Confectioner's sugar 1 cup

Instructions

1. Get a large bowl for mixing, then add in your granu-

lated sugar ½ cup, salt, baking powder, flour 1 cup, and finally, your shortening. Properly beat the mixture till your shortening is well integrated to form a mixture mirroring that of small pebbles.

2. Have your milk warmed to slightly above the average body temperature by having it heated inside a saucepan or preferably inside your microwave for a minute. Next, put in your vanilla paste, yeast, and sugar 1 tbsp. properly whisk the mixture and place aside.

3. After approximately five minutes of the mixture at rest, you'll notice that the mixture has begun rising as well as bubbling (presence of yeast) slowly stir it to your flour mixture together with the eggs (have your eggs first whisked before addition). Put in the remaining flour, a cup after another till your dough becomes firm but still slightly.

4. With your already cleaned countertop or a pastry mat, if you have one, flour it lightly then transfer your dough. Ensure to pat it properly, forming a disk shape (flat) then afterward carefully roll out all to a ½ inch thick.

5. The next step of making the donuts, flour your round cutter (large) and then have it pressed in your rolled dough. Using your preferred cookie cutters, out piece the middles.

6. Now on to the next step of engineering the holes, use a much smaller cookie cutter then gently and carefully press the scraps of your dough all together for re-cutting to ensure full use of the dough.

7. Now on making donut holes, roll every cut circle gently between your hands/palms till its ball-like in shape. After they have been cut and rolled, put your donuts on the baking sheet that has already been lined using parchment and as well cover using another parchment.

8. For the donuts now to rise, make sure to place them inside a warmer location, or instead, you could turn on your baking unit heated to 200 degrees F then turned off.

For Frying:

1. Get a large saucepan then put in your vegetable oil (2 inches), which you will heat to 350 degrees. Inside the saucepan, now add your donuts in a sequence of 3 or 4 at a go as you adjust and readjust your heat levels to maintain the oil temperature at 325 to 350 degrees.
2. With your donuts in the oil, have them fried till golden brown in color, off course flipping for an even browning and proper cooking. This being a fast cooking processing, it won't take you more than a minute, but be careful and keen not to undercook or overcook the yeasted donuts.
3. After you're sure, they are ready to remove them from the oil and place them on a wire rack for them to drain. If you opt to roll them in sugar, the ensure to do so when they are straight-up hot if you go the glazes way then allow your work of art to cool down first. Remove the cooked donuts using your slotted spoon then let it drain on a rack (wire).

Glaze:

1. For making the glaze, whisk all its ingredients into any sizable pan (sauce) over warm temperatures/ heat. Once it has warmed up well and integrated, dunk in your donuts and then place them aside onto your cooling rack, which ought to be covered using wax paper.
2. In terms of making the chocolate glaze, have all the essential ingredients whisked altogether till it is

thick but still able to be spread. Take your donuts and dip their tops in the glaze then as well place aside on the rack till it is all set (the glaze). For better consistency of your practice, you could add in some more milk or less of its right.

3. Now to get your donuts filled, as long as they are fried and well cooled, make sure to fit a sizable big opening icing tip (metal) inside your pastry bag, then fill it with preserves, jam, frosting or even cream as you're withdrawing the tip.

4. Keenly push the tip inside the interior side of your donut hole nearing the middle section and have your cram or jam generously squeezed inside.

5. In case of a larger sized donut, use a pastry bag well fixed with a longer tip in the middle then do just like the above instruction states.

PALEO CINNAMON ROLLS

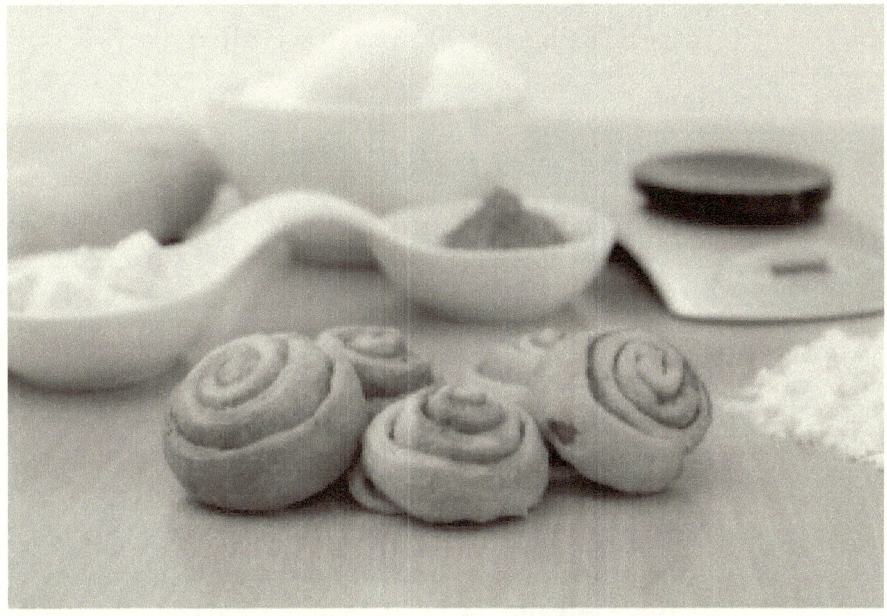

Preparation time to finishing time: 45 min

Ingredients:

- Macadamia nuts 2 cups
- Psyllium husks 2 tbsp. ground
- Coconut flour 8 tbsp.
- Grass-fed ghee 2 tbsp.
- Sweetened erythritol (monk fruit) 3 tbsp.
- Vanillas extract 2 tsp.
- Eggs 4
- Salt (a pinch)

- Ceylon cinnamon 3 tsp.

- Baking powder (paleo) 1 ½ tsp.

- Vinegar (apple cider) 1 tbsp.

- Caramel Sauce (keto) 1 batch & chilled

Glaze ingredients:

- Coconut cream 4 tbsp.

- Grass-fed ghee, 2 tbsp. & melted

- Birch xylitol 2 tsp. or erythritol

Instructions:

1. Using your blender or any food processor at your home, start by blending the macadamia nuts till they have a finer texture (before they turn to be too buttery). In such a case where it turns to be buttery, your cinnamon rolls won't be very fluffy but will still get baked.

2. Put together every cinnamon roll essential ingredients apart from the caramel sauce afterward, place them in the fridge to chill for about an hour.

3. Have your oven heated to temperatures of 350 degrees. On the side, ensure to line your baking tray using parchment.

4. On your parchment-lined countertop/surface, continue by rolling out the dough using your hands, forming a big rectangle.

5. Now pick a spoon and gently using its back spread the caramel sauce all over your batter, ensuring to spread close to its edges as possible.

6. Carefully roll your dough, forming a log then seal

its edge.

7. Take a sharp knife and have it warm in warm water. Afterward, since the dough logs to 10-12 equal rolls.

8. Putt each roll onto the lined tray then have them baked for approximately 25-30 min; in the process, remember to check after 20 min for readiness/doneness.

9. As your rolls are baking, it's the right time to have the glaze prepared. Take all the relevant ingredients and have them blended inside your mixing bowl or just until it combined adequately.

10. It's now time to remove your rolls from the baking unit/oven. Give them some time to cool off before you start glazing. Better yet, you could as well have them served warm with your glazed drizzled up top. In case of any leftovers or surplus pieces, ensure to cover and store in the fridge.

Produce: 10-12 pieces

Nutritional Information

Iron 1mg, calcium 52mg, vitamin D 5mcg, potassium 163mg, cholesterol 85mg, protein 5.6g, net carbs 5g, sugar alcohols 5g, total sugars 2.3g, dietary fiber 7.1g, sodium 127 mg, carbs 17.1mg, total fat 45.6mg, calories 477

Helpful Note on ingredients:

Apart from coconut, each and every nut is well considered a prime suspect when it comes to the bulletproof diet, all due to their high contents of fats (omega6) that oxidize and thereafter cause inflammation. Nuts themselves are prone to mold attack and as well contain lectins. These are basically nutrient sapping elements that could be tough all on your gut. So in the usage of nuts, be careful and moderate in their use or rather just get rid of them from any diet then much later in small quantities reintroduce them gradually to test body reactions.

PUMPKIN DONUTS

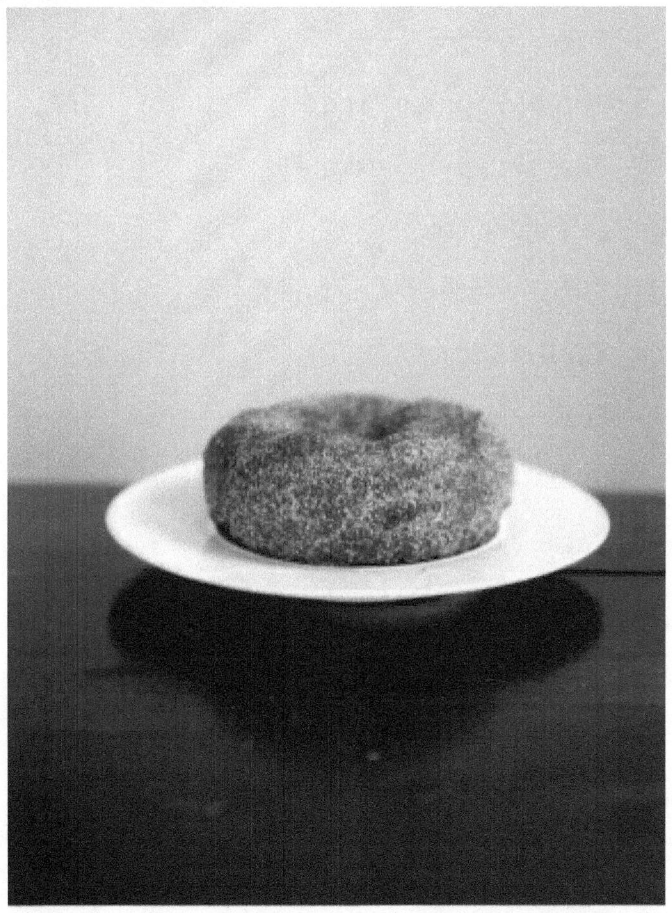

Imagine something soft, sweet that you can make in no time. Aren't pumpkin donuts just the best! No hassle, no long and tedious recipes. All tasty and healthy for just pastry!

The prepping time is 10 min, the cooking is time 15 min = total time 25 min

Essentials

For the donuts

- Vegetable oil ¼ cup

- 2 eggs

- Sugar ¾ cups

- Pumpkin puree ¾ cup

- Pumpkin pie spice one tsp.

- Salt half a tsp.

- Bicarbonate of soda one tsp.

- Vanilla ½ tsp.

- Flour one cup all-purpose

For the sugar coating

- Sugar 3 tbsp.

- Cinnamon 2 tsp.

Instructions

1. Have your oven heated to temperatures of 350 degrees.

2. Get your pan and have it sprayed using a nonstick spray.

3. Get the baking powder, pumpkin puree, vanilla, pumpkin pie spice, salt oil, and eggs and mix properly till well combined.

4. Stir in your flour as you continue mixing till it becomes smooth.

5. Get the donut pans and have them filled only ¾ ways to allow room for the rise.

6. Have your donuts baked for about 15-17 min.

7. After proper baking, remove them from your baking unit/oven. Allow them to cool down for about 5 minutes, then after that, remove them from the pan.

8. Take a large plastic bag and there in combine your cinnamon and sugar.

9. Carefully one after the other, place your donuts inside the bag and lightly shake to have the wholly immersed and covered.

10. After that, remove from the bag then allow then to cool off completely. For storage, an airtight container is considered best.

Essential Recipe Notes

This Recipe makes about (12) donuts-3 inch, or just (6) large ones. In case you love them Large and fleshy, you'll adjust your time to approximately 23-35 min.

CHOCOLATE COCONUT DONUTS

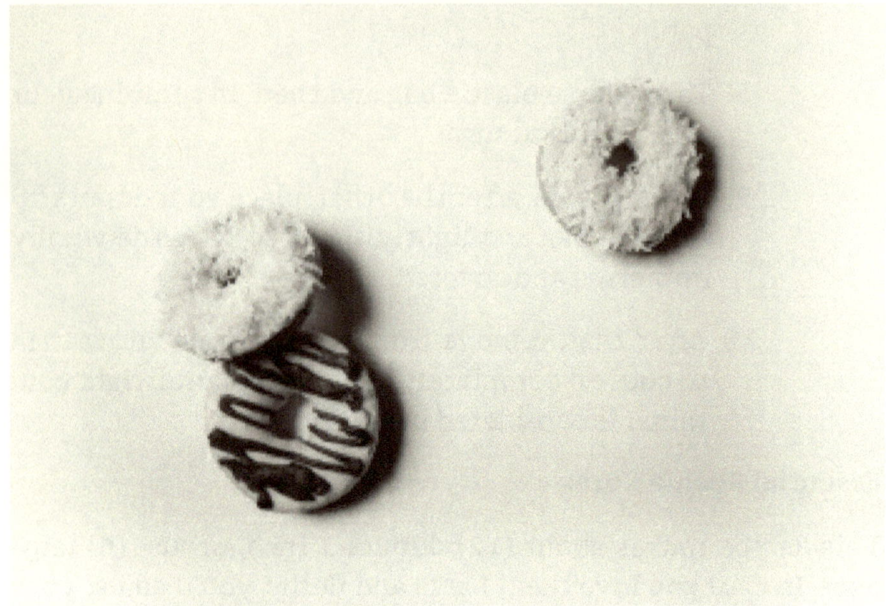

Prepping time of 10 min, the cooking time of 13 min = total time of 23 min

Servings of 14 pieces

Ingredients

- Eggs- 6 at room temp.

- Coconut flour ½ cup

- Lakanto White ½ cup or your preferred paleo or keto sweetener

- Cocoa powder ¼ cup

- Coconut oil ¼ cup softened/melted

- Coconut butter ¼ cup softened/melted

- Vanilla extract half a tsp.

- Teaspoon-a half coconut extract.

- Bicarbonate of soda half tsp.

- Half tsp. of baking soda

- Chocolate chips (Lilly's) ¾ cup or your preferred paleo chips

Coconut Butter Glaze & Chocolate Drizzle

- Coconut butter ½ cup & melted

- Vanilla stevia-liquid 4 drops (optional)

- Chocolate chips (Lilly's) ¼ cup & melted

- Coconut oil 1 tsp.

- Unsweetened coconut 3 tbsp. shredded (to garnish)

Instructions

Chocolate Coconut Donuts

1. Have your oven heated to 350 degrees as you grease your donut.

2. Take the cocoa powder, coconut oil, eggs, sweetener, coconut flour as well as coconut butter and carefully combine them in your mixing bowl. Properly do so till you obtain a smooth batter.

3. Into the same mixture, take the coconut extracts, vanilla, baking soda, and the baking powder and mix till well combined. You can either opt to dig in your hands and mix, or you can use your stand mixer.

4. The last thing, fold in the chocolate chips.

5. Transfer your donut batter into your bag zip-top (gallon-sized) with a ½" hole pierced into one corner.

6. Next pipe your donut batter in your donut pan (greased), filling every well till half-full.

7. Have it bake for 12-13 minutes.

8. Afterward, remove immediately then turn out on your cooling rack.

9. Repeat the filling process for each well, then baking till you've finished the batter.

Making the Drizzle

1. Put the coconut butter (melted) inside a bowl bigger than the donuts. If preferred, you can whisk in some drops of vanilla stevia.

2. Dip each donut's top into the coconut butter as you shake and tap gently, getting rid of any excess if preferred.

3. Sprinkle the unsweetened coconut (shredded) on every donut before your glaze sets.

4. Melt your chocolate chips & coconut oil (1 tsp.) over the double boiler.

5. As you would like it, drizzle or maybe have the chocolate dropped on every donut.

6. Have them stored inside an airtight container/bag or Store in an airtight container then refrigerate.

Nutrition Facts

1mg iron, 83mg calcium, vitamin A 40IU, protein 5g, sugar 10g, fiber 2g, carbs 23g, potassium 140mg, sodium 175mg, cholesterol 27mg, saturated fat 4g, fat 11g (daily value), 204 calories.

ALMOND FLOUR KETO DONUTS

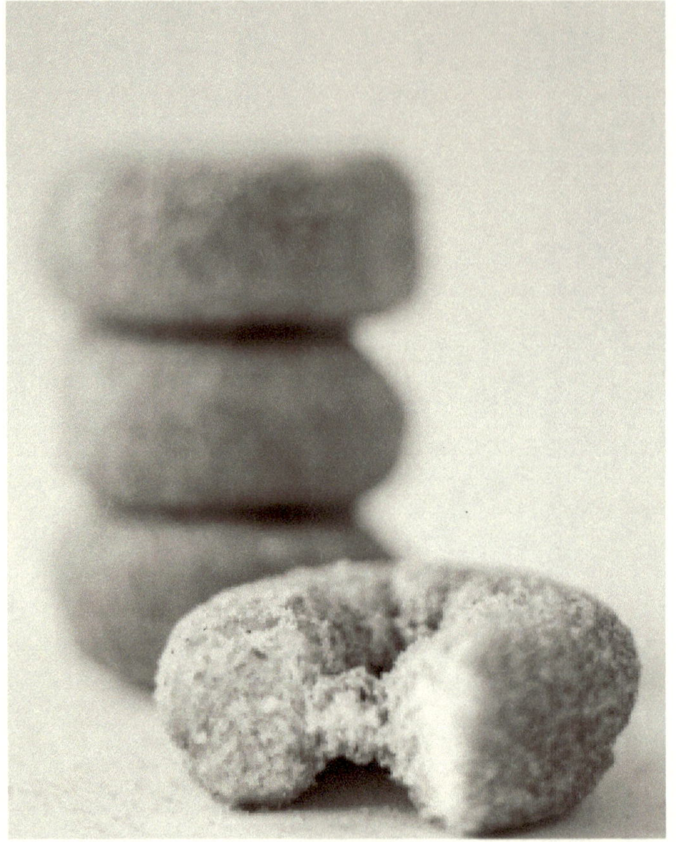

This is one very easy yet delicious donut recipe. With the sugar coating, it's all a burst of flavor into your taste buds.

Prepping Time: 15 min, Cooking Time: 25 min = total time: 40 min

Essentials

Donuts

- Flour-almond one cup (blanched)

- Erythritol a third a cup

- Baking powder 2 teaspoons. (gluten-free)

- Cinnamon 1 tsp.

- Sea salt 1/8 tsp.

- Butter ¼ cup (unsalted solid & melted)

- Almond milk ¼ cup (unsweetened)

- Egg 2 large

- Vanillas extract ½ tsp.

Cinnamon Coating

- Erythritol ½ cup

- Cinnamon 1 tsp.

- Butter 3 tbsp. (unsalted, solid & melted)

Instructions

1. Get the oven heated to 350degrees as you grease your donut pan in the meantime.

2. Using your large bowl, have the cinnamon, sea salt, baking powder, the almond flour, and erythritol mixed inside.

3. Take a relatively small bowl, then whisk all together with the eggs, almond milk, melted butter, plus your vanilla extract. Take your wet mixture whisk into your dry mixture.

4. Afterward, transfer your batter all evenly in the donut placed cavities, carefully filling each and one of them 3/4 full. Have it bake for 22-28 min (or a bit longer if you're using the silicone pan) till golden brown (dark). Allow it to cool till the donuts are

easily removable from the baking pan.

5. Meanwhile, inside another small bowl, take the erythritol as well as cinnamon and stir in for your coating.

6. After your donuts have properly cooled and easily removed from molds, have them transferred to your cutting board. Get both sides of your donuts brushed with butter, afterward roll/press into the cinnamon/sweetener mixture for coating. Do the same for all donut pieces.

Nutrition

1g sugar, 2g fiber, 5g carbs, 3g net carbs, 25g fat, 6g protein, 257 calories.

References

Pixie2016. (2019). Keto - Mozarella rolls stuffed with marinara, pepperoni, and jalapenos. Retrieved from https://www.copymethat.com/r/k9kzqPS/keto-mozarella-rolls-stuffed-with-marina/

Rege, L. (2019, August 7). Keto Cinnamon Rolls Recipe. Retrieved from https://www.delish.com/cooking/nutrition/a28541252/keto-cinnamon-rolls-recipe/

CHAPTER 9: HOW TO REDUCE WEIGHT USING KETO DIET (7 KG IN 5 DAYS)

Keto diet comprises of a lot of fats and proteins and low amounts of carbohydrates. Body cells prefer using blood glucose (blood sugar) to generate energy. Keto diet plays the role of forcing your body to adopt the use of new fuel.

The keto diet relies on the liver to breakdown fats into ketones. This is different from the usual norm where your body obtains energy by breaking down glucose from carbohydrates. The process of breaking down fat molecules into ketones is known as ketogenesis. Ketosis happens when fat becomes the primary source of energy in the body.

For the body to start using stored fat as fuel, one has to limit the carbohydrate he or she takes to about 20- 50 grams per day. The amount depends on the body size of the person. In some cases, the individual taking the diet may find themselves having to stick on a strict diet routine for the keto diet to have positive results in their system. Once an individual starts the keto diet, they can reach it in two to four days.

This is when 90% of your body starts depending on fats as the primary source of energy. Research has proven that it is easier to achieve weight loss using a keto diet than with the conventional calorie- reduction diet.

A keto diet is a safe form of weight loss. Also, those on the keto diet may find it a bit challenging to maintain the weight at the same level. The diet requires a lot of discipline in terms of how you take your diet.

Keto diet beginners should opt for healthier sources of fat and protein. Some of the sources include avocados, olive oil, nuts, almonds, and walnuts. After a month or so, you can switch to those foods with minimal amounts of fats. This will work better when you involve physical activities along.

Over time, the ketogenic diet is considered as the most effective weight-loss method. It not only reduces the amount of fat significantly from your body but also ensures that fat is kept off for good. Low carbohydrates and a high amount of protein will be effective after six months. At this period, your body has already adapted to the keto diet fully.

The keto diet comes with a set of rules to be followed, which makes it easier for one to resist the urge of overeating. The brain and the nervous system are some of the organs and body systems that benefit from the ketosis process.

When the human body starts to burn ketones as sources of fuel, the ketogenic dieters will have an increased energy level and a reduced appetite. This will translate to lesser consumption of calories, thus leading to weight loss. Water loss in the body happens during this period and contributes significantly to the reduced appetite and reduced use of calories.

The results of the keto diet are experienced and recorded a few days after one begins taking the diet. You are likely to lose 2-10 pounds during the first week of observing the keto diet. It is a significant milestone compared to other weight loss methods. However, all the glory should not only be given to fat but also the water loss that is a result of the process. The water lost during the process is a result of the body releasing the extra water it previously had as a result of the consumption of carbohydrate consumption.

After 2-3 weeks of the keto diet, the level of weight loss will reduce significantly and will be stable at a certain weight. In this period, the body shifts from relying on carbohydrates as a source of energy to fats. The average weight loss after the first two weeks will be 1-2 pounds per week.

You should also avoid taking snacks that are not in line with your dietary plans. One should stick to having at least two to three meals per day. Another option for fat fasting is observing intermittent fasting. This is merely restricting your meals within eight hours period. This will enable the levels of insulin and blood sugar to drop down to low levels. It will consequently help burn body fat for fuel.

One should avoid taking foods and drinks that they are allergic to. Keto diet does not go well with allergens. If your body finds it difficult to cope with gluten or dairy products, then you should avoid taking the products. Ensure your body is not stressed or fatigued. Too much exercise will not be suitable for your body due to a low metabolic rate.

Eating the right amount of protein will help the keto diet take effect smoothly in the body. However, taking too much protein will increase the levels of insulin in the body. This will reduce the amount of ketone in the body. Taking lesser amounts of protein will cause the body to burn muscle faster than fat. It is advisable to have daily exercises together with the right amount of proteins. With physical activities, the protein levels range around 0.8- 1.0g of protein.

Losing weight should not translate to muscle loss. The nutrient that is responsible for muscle building is protein. Proteins are essential when one is taking the keto diet. Ketones are known for preserving muscle tissues in the body. One should eat the right amount of protein for the keto diet to take effect in the body.

Taking a lot of protein will harm the body. This is because it will lower the amounts of ketosis in the body. To be sure that you are taking the right amount of protein, divide your protein into equal amounts, over the two to three meals. For those people that work out, they are advised to take more protein before and after work out to replenish the muscle tissues.

When observing the keto diet, it is essential to track the progress of your weight loss journey. You can measure the weight loss by recording the height, weight, and circumference of your body. This can help you estimate the weight loss of your body. The following steps will help you determine the level of weight loss:

- Tie the tape measure around your waist at the region where the belly button is located.

- Inhale and exhale a large amount of air and ensure the tape is well secured around the waist.

- Record the measurements and calculate the percentage of the fat in the body using the fat calculator.

- Repeat the procedure regularly at intervals of around two to three weeks to track down your progress.

The main reason why ketogenesis is effective is that it relies on whole foods like meat, low- carb vegetables, high- fat dairy, and enough amounts of protein. The main secret behind the success of the keto diet is in its consistency. For one to be sure that the ketogenesis is working in their body, the following steps and regulations should be taken:

- Ensure your body stress levels are low

- Exercise your body regularly but don't overdo it

- Lift weights. It is aimed at improving your body muscles

- You can adopt the fat fasting strategy to cut down the amount of fat in the body

- Take only the right amounts of food and avoid overeating.

Keto Diet and Improvement of the Skin

Having high amounts of oil in your food can make the skin look healthier. However, too much fat in the body can cause the skin to breakdown. This is caused by the increased production of sebum, which causes the skin to malfunction. The process may eventually cause acne. Diets that are rich in fats can lead to more skin inflammation in the body. It can also cause psoriasis.

Having high levels of insulin can worsen skin acne conditions. Keto diet will lower the skin acne condition. You should, however, avoid taking too much of the keto diet. High levels of ketones can lead to a skin condition called prurigo pigmentosa. This is a skin rash that is itchy and is visible around the back and chest region.

Keto diet mostly encourages the intake of fats that help reduce skin damage that comes from the sun. The diet has an impact on gut bacteria, which are essential to the growth of the hair, nails, and skin. Omega- 3 is suitable for the proper growth of hair and skin.

Keto diet is responsible for the improvement of your skin and weight loss. You can prove this by calculating your calorie needs every day and recording down the findings.

Keto diet users are advised to keep an open mind while observing weight loss. This is because weight loss is not consistent with all individuals. You might note during some weeks that you haven't lost any weight while in some weeks you have lost 3-4 pounds. What are some of the factors that contribute to how your body responds to weight loss on the keto diet?

- The health status of your body. The general health condition of the body affects the effectiveness of the keto diet. Having health conditions like resistance to insulin, having excess fat, and complication of the thyroid glands can affect how the keto diet takes effect in the body.

- The composition of your body. The body composition of individual humans determines the rate at which the keto diet will affect the body. Some individuals have a lot of fat in the body, while others do not have. The same case applies to muscle in the body. Those who have much fat in the body will tend to lose it faster than those with less amount of it. It is explained by the fact that those that are obese tend to exhibit a low-calorie deficit, which results in quick weight gain. The muscle mass of an individual will also contribute immensely to how the particular individual will lose weight. Muscle mass will help maintain the healthy body metabolic rate from dropping by a large proportion as one loses weight.

- Your day- to- day habit. Being on the keto diet requires one to be disciplined and have a lot of consistency for it to bear results. Ensure that you stick strictly to the keto diet and avoid any high- fat food that has low amounts of nutrients. The keto diet works very well with exercises. Taking the right food and at the right time, together with training, will lead to the successful transformation of the body.

- The amount of calorie lacking in your body. The body loses weight when you consume lesser amounts of calories than it requires. However, one should not stop taking the calories entirely as the body needs small amounts of calories as it loses some weight. The calorie deficit that is above 30% is considered to be unhealthy.

Keto Diet Always the most energetic combo

The primary function of ketosis is to burn body fats and converts fat into energy. The presence of ketones in the blood is a sign of ketosis. This can be easily tested using urine samples. Knowing what you eat is the key to a successful keto diet. When taking a keto diet, food is broken down in the following proportions; 75% fats, 20 % protein, and 5% carbohydrates.

The energy comes from the ketones- fuel molecules. When one is under the keto diet, they should avoid taking food that is rich in carbs, starch, and sugar. This means that you should not take food that is rich in starch, such as bread, pasta, rice, or potatoes. You should take an average of 30- 150 grams of carbs in a single day. Keto diet is generally safe for most people.

However, one should watch out for the possibility of side effects such as dehydration and muscle cramps, insomnia, and lack of sleep. Ensure your keto diet comes from leafy sources such as vegetables and fiber-rich kales. One should also take at least 2 ½ of salt per day to retain sufficient water to keep the bowels regular.

Keto diet users have the liberty to decide how much fat they want in their body. However, achieving the results of this diet requires a lot of consistency, discipline, and a well- planned dietary approach. To be on the right path for your keto journey, you should be on the watch out for the following fundamental principles:

- Always take the correct amount of protein and calories to help you achieve your dietary goals.

- You can obtain calories from micronutrient dense foods.

- Ensure that the diet works for you. If, after two to three weeks, you do not observe anything positive, then you should consult your keto diet expert for them to advise accordingly.

- Adjust your lifestyle for it to create an enabling environment for the keto diet to work well.

After two weeks of using the keto diet, you should observe the following body parameters for any changes:

- The general mood and well-being of your body

- The body composition

- The amounts of ketone in your body

- The levels of different body markers. These include cholesterol, blood- sugar levels, and blood pressure).

People who are on a keto diet are advised to try fat fast. It happens when you take low amounts of fat and calories for three days. It will increase the burning of fat in the body. The energy is distributed across the body in accordance with the needs of the body systems.

References

Clarke, C. (2019, September 13). How to Lose Weight on a Ketogenic Diet [Blog post]. Retrieved from https://www.ruled.me/how-to-lose-weight-ketogenic-diet/

Perfect Keto. (n.d.). How to Use the Ketogenic Diet for Weight Loss [Blog post]. Retrieved from https://perfectketo.com/use-ketogenic-diet-weight-loss/

CONCLUSION

Thank you very much for having read this book. It is my greatest hope that the book is highly informative and educative. The book, 'Keto Bread' introduces you to the world of weight loss. Many people around the globe are struggling with health-related complications such as obesity, among others. Keto Bread comes in handy with rich information and guidelines on how to lose weight using ketogenic products. The book has a precious message sandwiched with practical that, when implemented correctly, you will be in a position to lose almost 7 kg within five days. As far as much has been mentioned in the previous chapters, it is well evident that this book suits everyone. That's, people who feel they can't lose weight will automatically shed off some pounds, and within the long run, they will be much thinner. Another target group is those who fail to train but would wish to lead a good life. They have the best book here that if they implement it, then they will be able to lose weight quickly. The book targets almost everyone within the sphere since it provides an excellent foundation where you eat and get filled up, but at the end of the day, you are losing some weight.

The Keto Bread book initiates you into the process of ketosis, which is a state of metabolism. It is through this process that the body can yield energy using fats. However, to know much about this, it will be better to concentrate more on these chapters talking much about ketosis. Again, keto flu and all the products that are allowed in this process. Still, for you to undergo the full process of ketosis so that you lose weight while eating, you need to know the products that you are supposed to avoid in this diet.

No one hates sweet and savory meals. However, in most cases, these are considered as ingredients that increase body weight. In keto diet, there are sweet and savory recipes with less carb, moderate protein, and high-fat content that will still give you the best feeling ever. It is my hope that you will still go back and take a look at them.

Cooking different muffins, cookies, rolls, buns, fat bombs, donuts, and other keto products has been made easier. That's, there is the availability of these ingredients within our area of disposal. In most cases, the keto diet uses low carb flours and sweeteners that will help in weight reduction. The keto Bread book is mainly for weight loss even though the various products used are very beneficial, especially in treating skin defects. More so, these products can reduce heart-related risks.

The book, Keto Bread, has eventually achieved more than what has been written. Using this book will enable you to lose weight quickly even without going to the gym, doing strenuous exercises, or being subjected to medication. Fortunately, the book is also helpful in treating heart-related diseases such as blood sugar level, hypertension, insulin level, and even cholesterol level.

Therefore, if you want to lose weight within five days, then this book is the best choice. Within the book, there are several great recipes that will help you make your ketogenic diets. You can do as much exercise as you can until you get to your best level.

Hoping that the book has been helpful and you will implement everything that has been written here, I would like to ask for your humble request. In any case, you will have some extra time, don't hesitate to make reviews on other sites since when essential information like this is shared, it will help solve a problem.